# Assessment of Future Scientific Needs for

# Live Variola Virus

Committee on the Assessment of Future Scientific Needs for
Live Variola Virus

Board on Global Health

INSTITUTE OF MEDICINE

NATIONAL ACADEMY PRESS
Washington, D.C. 1999

NATIONAL ACADEMY PRESS • 2101 Constitution Avenue, N.W. • Washington, D.C. 20418

NOTICE: The project that is the subject of this report was approved by the Governing Board of the National Research Council, whose members are drawn from the councils of the National Academy of Sciences, the National Academy of Engineering, and the Institute of Medicine. The members of the committee responsible for the report were chosen for their special competences and with regard for appropriate balance.

The Institute of Medicine was chartered in 1970 by the National Academy of Sciences to enlist distinguished members of the appropriate professions in the examination of policy matters pertaining to the health of the public. In this, the Institute acts under both the Academy's 1863 congressional charter responsibility to be an adviser to the federal government and its own initiative in identifying issues of medical care, research, and education. Dr. Kenneth I. Shine is president of the Institute of Medicine.

This study was supported by the U.S. Department of Defense, the U.S. Department of Energy, and the U.S. Department of Health and Human Services. The views presented in this report are those of the Institute of Medicine Committee on the Assessment of the Future Need for Variola (Smallpox) Virus and are not necessarily those of the funding agencies.

Additional copies of this report are available for sale from the National Academy Press, Box 285, 2101 Constitution Avenue, N.W., Washington, D.C., 20055. Call (800) 624-6242 or (202) 334-3313 (in the Washington metropolitan area), or visit the NAP online bookstore at **www.nap.edu**.

The complete text of *Assessment of Future Scientific Needs for Live Variola Virus* is available on line at **www.nap.edu**.

For more information about the Institute of Medicine, visit the IOM home page at **www4.nas.edu/IOM/IOMHome.nsf**.

Copyright 1999 by the National Academy of Sciences. All rights reserved.

Printed in the United States of America.

COVER: Bio-Safety Level 4 Containment Laboratory at U.S. Army Medical Research Institute of Infectious Diseases, Fort Detrick, Maryland. Copyright Brian R. Wolff / IIPI. All rights reserved.

## COMMITTEE ON THE ASSESSMENT OF FUTURE NEEDS FOR VARIOLA (SMALLPOX) VIRUS

**CHARLES C. J. CARPENTER** (*Chair*), Brown University International Health Institute, Providence, Rhode Island
**ANN M. ARVIN,** Stanford University School of Medicine, Palo Alto, California
**R. PALMER BEASLEY,** University of Texas-Houston Health Science Center School of Public Health
**KENNETH I. BERNS,** University of Florida College of Medicine, Gainesville
**RAPHAEL DOLIN,** Harvard University Medical School, Boston, Massachusetts
**MYRON E. ESSEX,** Harvard School of Public Health, Boston, Massachusetts
**DIANE E. GRIFFIN,** Johns Hopkins University School of Public Health, Baltimore, Maryland
**ASHLEY T. HAASE,** University of Minnesota Medical School, Minneapolis
**MARTIN S. HIRSCH,** Harvard University Medical School, Boston, Massachusetts
**ELLIOTT KIEFF,** Harvard University and Brigham and Women's Hospital, Boston, Massachusetts
**PETER S. KIM,** Whitehead Institute for Biomedical Research and Massachusetts Institute of Technology, Cambridge, Massachusetts
**BERNARD LO,** University of California at San Francisco Program in Medical Ethics
**D. GRANT MCFADDEN,** Robarts Research Institute, London, Ontario, Canada
**BERNARD MOSS,** National Institute for Allergy and Infectious Diseases, National Institutes of Health, Bethesda, Maryland
**RICHARD W. MOYER,** University of Florida College of Medicine, Gainesville
**HIDDE L. PLOEGH,** Harvard University Medical School and Free University of Amsterdam, Netherlands
**JACK SCHMIDT,** Merck Research Laboratories, Rahway, New Jersey
**RICHARD J. WHITLEY,** University of Alabama at Birmingham Children's Hospital
**FLOSSIE WONG-STAAL,** University of California at San Diego School of Medicine

*Staff*

**JUDITH R. BALE,** Director, Board on Global Health
**ROB COPPOCK,** Study Consultant
**STACEY L. KNOBLER,** Research/Administrative Assistant
**STEPHANIE BAXTER-PARROTT,** Project Assistant
**RONA BRIERE,** Editor

## BOARD ON GLOBAL HEALTH

**BARRY R. BLOOM** (*Cochair*), Harvard University School of Public Health, Boston, Massachusetts
**DEAN JAMISON** (*Cochair*), University of California at Los Angeles and the World Health Organization, Geneva, Switzerland
**JACQUELYN CAMPBELL,** Johns Hopkins University School of Nursing, Baltimore, Maryland
**HARVEY V. FINEBERG,** Harvard University, Cambridge, Massachusetts
**JULIO FRENK,** World Health Organization, Geneva, Switzerland
**EILEEN T. KENNEDY,** Research, Education, and Economics, U.S. Department of Agriculture, Washington, D.C.
**ARTHUR KLEINMAN,** Harvard Medical School, Boston, Massachusetts
**BERNARD LIESE,** The World Bank, Washington, D.C.
**WILLIAM E. PAUL,** National Institute of Allergy and Infectious Diseases and Office of AIDS Research, National Institutes of Health, Bethesda, Maryland
**ALLAN ROSENFIELD,** Columbia University School of Public Health, New York, New York
**PATRICIA L. ROSENFIELD,** The Carnegie Corporation of New York, New York
**THOMAS J. RYAN,** Boston University School of Medicine and Boston University Medical Center, Massachusetts
**JUNE E. OSBORN** (*Institute of Medicine Liaison*), Josiah Macy, Jr., Foundation, New York, New York
**DAVID R. CHALLONER** (*Institute of Medicine Foreign Secretary*), Institute for Science and Health Policy, University of Florida, Gainesville

*Staff*

**JUDITH R. BALE,** Director
**STACEY L. KNOBLER,** Research/Administrative Assistant
**STEPHANIE BAXTER-PARROTT,** Project Assistant
**KAY HARRIS,** Financial Associate

◆ ◆ ◆ ◆ ◆ ◆

# Preface

The global eradication of smallpox stands as the most successful public health campaign in medical history. Smallpox was one of the most feared of plagues, the very epitome of the dread associated with rampant and devastating illness. Its eradication required the cooperation of dedicated physicians, public health officials, governments, and untold individuals around the world. Once that goal had been accomplished, known materials containing variola virus, the pathogen responsible for smallpox, were consolidated in two international repositories.

It has been proposed by the World Health Organization that the two remaining stocks of variola be destroyed in June 1999. Advances in microbiology, however, now raise the question of the possible utility of retaining the only pathogenic virus humanity has been able to eradicate. The primary reason for the proposed destruction of the remaining known variola stocks is that, despite any medical advances that might result from studies using the live variola virus, the risks of retaining and working with the virus (ranging from accidental laboratory release to acquisition and use by terrorists) may outweigh the benefits.

The U.S. Department of Defense, the U.S. Department of Energy, and the U.S. Department of Health and Human Services asked the Institute of Medicine to assess the scientific and medical information that might be lost were live variola virus no longer available for research purposes. The scientific and medical assessment presented in this report is but one of a number of efforts aimed at examining various aspects of the issue. The committee assembled to conduct this assessment includes not only those whose training and research gives them detailed knowledge of poxviruses, the class of organisms to which variola virus belongs, but also those whose background ensures consideration of broader medical and biological concerns. Also among the committee members are physicians who personally witnessed the devastation of smallpox prior to its eradication.

It is important to note that the committee was not asked to assess the likelihood that an outbreak of smallpox might occur as the result of accidental or intentional action or biological terrorism. In assessing future scientific needs for variola virus, however, the committee addressed questions likely to be directed to scientists should this pathogen be used as a terrorist weapon.

The committee assembled information from a variety of sources and in November 1998 conducted a public workshop attended by many of the nation's leading experts in fields related to the committee's charge. The workshop reviewed recent research on antiviral agents and vaccines, the status of detection and diagnosis technologies, and ways in which study of the variola virus might contribute to understanding of viral pathogenesis and the human immune system, and other research related to variola virus. This information was used by the committee to develop its findings and conclusions in meetings immediately following the November workshop and in January 1999.

This final report is addressed to health policymakers, medical and biological researchers, and the public as the committee's assessment of the knowledge that might be lost if live variola virus were no longer available for research.

Charles C. J. Carpenter
*Chair*

◆ ◆ ◆ ◆ ◆ ◆

# Acknowledgments

The committee appreciates the contributions of many individuals to this report. We express our gratitude to the experts who made presentations at the initial workshop: Mark Buller, Joseph Esposito, Donald A. Henderson, John Huggins, Peter Jahrling, Wolfgang Joklik, Sergei Shchelkunov, and Alan Zelicoff. We also thank the workshop participants who contributed their insights and raised important questions at the workshop.

The following agencies and key staff provided funding and generated support within their instititions for this study: the U.S. Department of Defense (Michael Fitzgibbon, Sally Horn, Frank Miller, Stephen Morse), the U.S. Department of Energy (Page Stoutland), and the U.S. Department of Health and Human Services (Margaret Hamburg, Robert Knouss, William Raub, Kevin Tonat). Their willingness to sponsor this study on variola virus is a significant commitment, given the sensitive and controversial nature of policy discussions surrounding broader issues involving the variola virus stocks. Kenneth Bernard, National Security Council staff, provided useful information on the broader context in which the report findings would be used.

The committee also thanks Stacey Knobler and Stephanie Baxter-Parrott for their excellent coordination of the committee's meetings and of the production this report, Rob Coppock for providing text for the committee's consideration, Rona Briere for editing the report, and Judith Bale for overall organization and execution of the effort.

This report has been reviewed in draft form by individuals chosen for their diverse perspectives and technical expertise, in accordance with procedures approved by the National Research Council's Report Review Committee. The purpose of this independent review is to provide candid and critical comments that will assist the Institute of Medicine in making the published report as sound as possible, and to ensure that the report meets institutional standards for objectivity, evidence, and responsiveness to the study charge. The review comments and draft manuscript remains confidential to protect the integrity of the deliberative process. The committee wishes to thank the following individuals for their participation in the review of this report:

## REVIEWERS

**RAFI AHMED,** Emory University Vaccine Center, Atlanta, Georgia
**ENRIQUETA BOND,** Burroughs Wellcome Fund, Durham, North Carolina
**MARK BULLER,** St. Louis University Medical School, Missouri
**ERIK DE CLERCQ,** Rega Institute for Medical Research, Leuven, Belgium
**KEITH DUMBELL,** University of London, United Kingdom
**JOSEPH ESPOSITO,** Centers for Disease Control and Prevention, Atlanta, Georgia
**FRANK FENNER,** John Curtain School of Medical Research, Australian National University, Canberra
**DON GANEM,** University of California at San Francisco
**ANNE GERSHON,** Columbia University College of Physicians and Surgeons, New York, New York
**DONALD A. HENDERSON,** Center for Civilian Biodefense Studies, The Johns Hopkins University, Baltimore, Maryland
**WOLFGANG JOKLIK,** Duke University, Durham, North Carolina
**JOSHUA LEDERBERG,** Rockefeller University, New York, New York
**JUNE OSBORN,** Josiah Macy, Jr., Foundation, New York, New York
**BERNARD ROIZMAN,** The University of Chicago, Illinois
**SIR JOHN SKEHEL,** National Institute for Medical Research, London, United Kingdom
**GEOFFREY SMITH,** Oxford University, Oxford, United Kingdom
**PATRICIA SPEAR,** Northwestern University Medical School, Chicago, Illinois
**MORTON SWARTZ,** Massachusetts General Hospital, Boston, Massachusetts
**ROLF ZINKERNAGEL,** University Hospital of Zurich and the Institute of Experimental Immunology, Zurich, Switzerland

We also wish to thank the following individuals for their review of technical portions of the report: John Becher and Joseph Esposito, Centers for Disease Control and Prevention, Atlanta; and John Huggins and Peter Jahrling, United States Army Medical Research Institute of Infectious Diseases, Fort Detrick, Maryland.

While the individuals listed above have provided constructive comments and suggestions, it must be emphasized that responsibility for the final content of this report rests entirely with the authoring committee and the Institute of Medicine.

# Contents

**EXECUTIVE SUMMARY** ............................................................................ 1

### PART I. INTRODUCTION

1 **Introduction** ........................................................................................ 7
   Background, 8
   Contemporary Context, 10
   Scope, 11
   Scientific Needs for Variola Virus, 11
   Organization of This Report, 13

### PART II. SMALLPOX AND ITS CONTROL

2 **Variola Virus and Other Orthopoxviruses** ............................................ 17
   General Attributes of Orthopoxviruses, 18
   Poxvirus Replication, 19
   Properties of Specific Orthopoxviruses, 20

3 **Clinical Features of Smallpox** ............................................................ 25
   Entry and Infection, 25
   Dissemination, 26
   The Rash, 27
   Lesions of the Mucous Membranes, 27
   Effects on Other Organs, 28
   Immune Response, 28
   Immunity Against Smallpox, 30

## 4 Epidemiology .................................................................................................. 33
Characteristics of Historical Outbreaks, 33
Likely Characteristics of Future Smallpox Outbreaks, 34
Control Strategies, 35

## 5 Variola Virus Stocks Following Eradication of Smallpox ...................... 37
Establishment of International Repositories, 38
Decision by the World Health Assembly to Destroy Variola
  Virus Stocks, 40
U.S. Research on Smallpox, 41
Research at CDC and USAMRIID, 42

# PART III. SCIENTIFIC NEEDS FOR VARIOLA VIRUS

## 6 Development of Antiviral Agents ............................................................. 47
In Vitro Assays, 48
Animal Models, 50

## 7 Development of Vaccines .......................................................................... 53
Current Status of Vaccinia Vaccine Preparations, 54
Evaluation of Vaccinia Vaccine Derived from Tissue Culture, 55
Evaluation of Novel Vaccines, 57

## 8 Detection and Diagnosis ............................................................................ 59
Environmental Detection, 60
Diagnosis of Infection, 61
Alternatives to Live Virus, 62

## 9 Bioinformatics ............................................................................................ 63
Variability of Variola Virus, 64
Potential Developments, 66

## 10 Understanding of the Biology of Variola Virus ..................................... 69
Virus-Cell Interactions, 69
Virus-Host Interactions, 70

## 11 Research on the Expressed Protein Products of Variola ...................... 73
Synthesis of Variola Proteins, 74
Potential Utility of Variola Proteins, 75

## PART IV. FINDINGS

**12 Summary and Conclusions** ................................................................... 79
The Broader Context, 80
Scientific Needs for Live Variola Virus, 81
Overall Conclusions, 85

**REFERENCES** ............................................................................................ 87

**APPENDIXES**
A  Glossary, 93
B  Acronyms, 99
C  Committee and Staff Biographies, 101

# Assessment of Future Scientific Needs for

## *Live Variola Virus*

❖ ❖ ❖ ❖ ❖ ❖

# Executive Summary

Smallpox is a devastating disease with high case-fatality and transmission rates. It is caused by variola, a large and complex virus from the orthopoxvirus family. In 1980, after millennia of suffering and death, smallpox was formally declared eradicated as the result of an intense worldwide program of inoculation with vaccinia virus.

Because scientific research on live variola virus has been restricted to maximum containment facilities in two international repositories, few research efforts have been undertaken using the live virus since eradication. During that time, scientific knowledge about the molecular pathogenesis of viral infections has become considerably more sophisticated. Variola virus is the only uniquely human orthopoxvirus, and exhibits a complex and well-tuned adaptation to exploit and circumvent the human immune system. Research using variola therefore offers the potential to contribute to mankind's knowledge of the human body's uniquely evolved system of defense against infection.

## SCOPE

In preparation for international deliberations concerning whether to destroy all known variola virus stocks, stored clinical materials containing live variola virus, and variola virus intact genome DNA held in the two international repositories, this committee was asked to assess future scientific needs for live variola virus. The committee's charge was restricted to that assessment. It did not include consideration of risks that may be associated with retention of the existing stocks, and no attempt was made to determine whether the scientific needs identified by the committee outweigh these risks. Furthermore, the committee did not address the likelihood that the funds and other resources needed to pursue this research, including facilities with suitable biological containment provisions, would be available. It must also be recognized that predicting the future is impossible, and while the committee has done its best to provide an assessment of future scientific needs for live variola virus, the unfolding of actual needs and opportunities is likely to depend on the emergence of unforeseeable technical developments, experimental tools, and model systems. For these reasons, the committee expresses its findings and conclusions below in conditional form: If particular knowledge or capability were to be pursued, would the associated research require live variola virus?

## SCIENTIFIC NEEDS FOR LIVE AND REPLICATION-DEFECTIVE VARIOLA VIRUS

The committee first notes a need associated with the short-term use of variola virus stocks.

**Genomic sequencing and limited study of variola surface proteins derived from geographically dispersed specimens is an essential foundation for important future work. Such research could be carried out now, and could require a delay in the destruction of known stocks, but would not necessitate their indefinite retention.**

Although some insight into variation might be obtained by restriction fragment length polymorphism comparison of variola genes amplified by polymerase chain reaction, the precise nature of individual gene variation and resultant impact on the protein product(s) requires more detailed sequencing. Given that the current policy is to destroy the stocks of variola virus in 1999, this need is urgent.

The committee identified six areas of research related to the potential scientific needs for live variola virus, replication-defective variola virus, and gene segments of variola virus.

**1. The most compelling reason for long-term retention of live variola virus stocks is their essential role in the identif-ication and development of antiviral agents for use in anticipation of a large outbreak of smallpox. It must be emphasized that if the search for antiviral agents with activity against live variola virus were to be continued, additional public resources would be needed.**

There is currently no effective antiviral for the treatment or prevention of variola. Only vaccination can reduce the severity of the disease, and only if administered within 4 days of exposure. The possibility of obtaining misleading results with surrogate viruses means that candidate antiviral agents must be tested against several clinical isolates of variola. Since smallpox has been eradicated, cell culture assays using live variola provide the only pre-outbreak opportunity to evaluate quantitatively the ability to block infection of (or replication within) human cells.

**2. Adequate stocks of smallpox vaccine must be maintained if research is to be conducted on variola virus or if maintenance of a smallpox vaccination program is required. Live variola virus would be necessary if certain approaches to the development of novel types of smallpox vaccine were pursued.**

Supplies of vaccinia vaccine in the United States have dwindled and may be deteriorating. In addition, vaccinia vaccine, which is used for smallpox immunization, is a live virus and cannot be used safely with immunocompromised individuals. This latter concern suggests a need for novel vaccines. Vaccines derived from tissue culture could be compared with the standard vaccine by evaluation in human subjects and by laboratory assays. Live variola virus would be required only for testing of novel vaccine development strategies using materials other than live vaccinia virus.

**3. If further development of procedures for the environmental detection of variola virus or for diagnostic purposes were to be pursued, more extensive knowledge of the genome variability, predicted protein sequences, virion surface structure, and functionality of variola virus from widely dispersed geographic sources would be needed.**

Evaluation of the specificity and sensitivity of detection methods for variola virus and other orthopoxviruses would require increased knowledge regarding the DNA sequence not only of variola virus from multiple geographic locations, but also of other orthopoxviruses, especially monkeypox.

**4. The existence of animal models would greatly assist the development and testing of antiviral agents and vaccines, as well as studies of variola pathogenesis. Such a program could be carried out only with live variola virus.**

The current absence of suitable animal models for variola virus does not mean that such models cannot be developed in the future, given advances in reconstituting certain experimental animals with human genes. There is no way of anticipating, however, when such a model system might become available.

**5. Live or replication-defective variola virus would be needed if studies of variola pathogenesis were to be undertaken to provide information about the response of the human immune system.**

The specific spatial and temporal patterns of variola virus gene expression must be deciphered in the context of infection at the level of cells, organs, and animal models. Studies of these phenomena could provide information on how the virus manipulates the human immune response in order to spread, on the mechanisms of cell death, and on other aspects of variola infection.

**6. Variola virus proteins have potential as reagents in studies of human immunology. Live variola virus would be needed for this purpose only until sufficient variola isolates had been cloned and sequenced.**

Variola virus could serve as a resource for the discovery of human-specific reagents, such as cytokine inhibitors, antiinflammatory proteins, and regulators of apoptosis.

## OVERALL CONCLUSIONS

The most compelling need for long-term retention of live variola virus is for the development of antiviral agents or novel vaccines to protect against a reemergence of smallpox due to accidental or intentional release of variola virus. In addition, much scientific information, particularly concerning the human immune system, could be learned through experimentation with live variola virus.

# PART I
♦ ♦ ♦ ♦ ♦

# Introduction

# 1
♦ ♦ ♦ ♦ ♦

# Introduction

Smallpox is a devastating disease with high case-fatality and transmission rates. It is caused by variola, a large and complex virus from the orthopoxvirus family, which infects only humans. A disease resembling smallpox has been described in many human populations over the last 3,000 years. In 1980, after millennia of suffering and death, variola virus was finally eradicated by a worldwide program of immunization with the related vaccinia virus.

The global eradication of this rampant and devastating disease, stands as the most successful campaign in medical history. Led by a major World Health Organization (WHO) program, it required the cooperation of governments, public health officials, physicians, and untold individuals in almost every country of the world. Once smallpox had been eradicated, all known materials containing variola virus, the responsible pathogen, were consolidated into two international repositories. The WHO Committee on Orthopoxvirus Infections subsequently voted to destroy all variola virus stocks, all stored clinical materials containing variola virus, and all intact variola virus DNA held in the international repositories in June 1999. Since this decision will be reconsidered in May 1999, the Institute of Medicine was asked to assess future scientific needs for live variola virus. This report is intended to serve health policymakers, medical and biological researchers, and the public as an assessment of the potential knowledge and capabilities that would be lost if live variola virus were no longer available for research purposes.

## BACKGROUND

Any assessment of the scientific needs for variola virus must include some grasp of the ravages of smallpox and the terrible suffering caused by the disease.

The incubation period of smallpox, which can be as short as 7 days or as long as 19 days, is a period of intense activity in terms of viral replication and spread within the body despite the absence of clinical symptoms. The incubation period ends when the patient becomes feverish and ill. The onset of fever is sudden, the patient's temperature usually rising to between 38.5°C and 40.5°C. Other symptoms include severe headache and backache. Vomiting occurs in about half and diarrhea in about 10 percent of cases. The patient frequently exhibits general lethargy and malaise. By the second or third day the temperature falls, and the patient feels somewhat better. At this time the smallpox rash begins to appear.

The lesions typically begin as minute red spots on the tongue and palate. Over a period of 24–48 hours, a macular rash appears on the face, then spreads to the trunk and extremities. The lesions progress over a 2-week period to vesicles, pustules, and crusts (scabs). A hemorrhagic and rapidly fatal form of the disease occurs in a minority of patients. Secondary infection of lesions can lead to osteomyelitis and septic arthritis, resulting in bone shortening, flail joints, and gross bone deformities. Scarred lesions or pockmarks remain with those who have survived the disease.

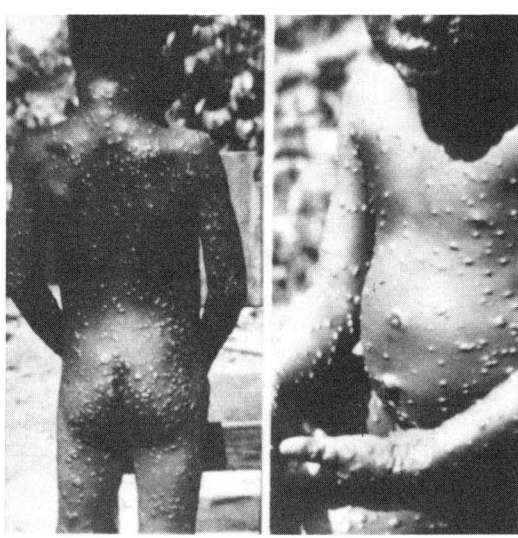

**PLATE 1.** Photos from the reverse of the WHO smallpox recognition card showing variola major pustules at their maximum size [1].

## INTRODUCTION

Smallpox is readily transmitted, with each patient typically infecting three or four others who have been in close contact [1]. Besides the characteristic eruptions, some patients have generalized collapse with failure of multiple organs during the initial stages of fever. However, patients are not infectious until the focal eruptions appear in the throat and on the skin.

A disease resembling smallpox was described as early as 1122 B.C. in China and is referred to in ancient Sanskrit texts of India. The Pharaoh Ramses V apparently died of smallpox in 1157 B.C. The disease spread from Japan and Korea and reached Europe in 710 A.D., and was transferred to America by Hernando Cortez in 1520; 3.5 million Aztecs died in the next 2 years. In cities of 18th-century Europe, smallpox reached plague proportions. Five reigning European monarchs died from smallpox during the 18th century [2, 3].

From the time it was first recognized until about the end of the 19th century, smallpox was regarded as a uniformly severe disease associated with a high case-fatality rate. However, starting about 1900 a less severe form of smallpox (variola minor) was recognized, exhibiting case-fatality rates of 1 percent or less in unvaccinated persons. During the first half of the 20th century, all outbreaks of smallpox in Asia and most of those in Africa were due to variola major, with case-fatality rates of 20 percent or more, while variola minor with case-fatality rates of 1 percent or less was endemic in some countries of Europe and North and South America. After the global smallpox eradication program was begun by WHO in 1959, more careful examination revealed some outbreaks in central and eastern Africa and in Indonesia with case-fatality rates of between 5 and 15 percent, but with clinical characteristics indistinguishable from those of variola major [1].

Although eradication of smallpox was established as a goal of WHO in 1959, preoccupation with malaria on the part of WHO and many member countries resulted in a relative lack of interest in smallpox until 1967, when the Intensified Smallpox Eradication Program was established. A strategic plan was developed, involving first mass vaccination, and then surveillance and containment of outbreaks [1].

The eradication of smallpox constituted, in principle, a straightforward disease control activity. An easily administered vaccine provided long-term protection. The presence of smallpox could be readily determined because of its distinctive rash. Only patients with a rash transmitted the infection to others, and then only to persons with whom they were in close contact. Because about 2 weeks elapsed before the infected person could transmit the disease to others, epidemics did not spread rapidly. Little more was required than to isolate the patient and vaccinate his or her close contacts. Nevertheless, global eradication of smallpox was a complex and difficult task that in the end required the cooperation of all countries. Famine, flood, epidemic cholera, and civil war all disrupted smallpox eradication efforts. Ultimately, a massive effort that effectively surveyed every household in countries where smallpox remained endemic was required to identify remaining cases and reduce the incidence of smallpox. The last naturally occurring case occurred on October 26, 1977, in Somalia, and in 1980 the World Health Assembly declared that smallpox had been eradicated [1].

## CONTEMPORARY CONTEXT

A smallpox outbreak today would present unique epidemiological and clinical features. Because smallpox vaccination ceased following eradication, an outbreak would occur in a population with little immunity, and therefore would differ substantially from other 20$^{th}$-century outbreaks of the disease. An outbreak today in a highly mobile and susceptible population would likely spread widely before being recognized and before appropriate countermeasures could be put in place. In addition, existing smallpox vaccines are not safe for use by individuals with compromised immune systems. Such individuals include those with AIDS (which emerged after smallpox was eradicated), those taking drugs designed to suppress rejection of organ transplants, and those being treated for cancer, all of whose numbers have grown tremendously. Finally, aerosolized variola virus is considered a serious threat as a biological weapon. Testimony before a committee of the U.S. Congress, for example, alleged that scientists in the former Soviet Union experimented with variola virus as a biological weapon on a large scale [4].

The possibility of a smallpox outbreak poses particular ethical and policy dilemmas regarding the retention of live variola virus stocks. Whether continued existence of such stocks would produce human benefits and reduce potential harm depends, in part, on whether the known stocks in the two tightly controlled international repositories are in fact the only remaining samples. While there are many potential medical advances that could derive from studies using live variola virus, the risks of maintaining and working with the virus (ranging from release due to laboratory accidents to acquisition and use by terrorists) may outweigh the benefits. Moreover, assessment of the benefits and risks of destroying or maintaining virus stocks may depend on regional and cultural factors. For example, a country that has suffered recent outbreaks of smallpox may make a different assessment than a nation that has been relatively free of smallpox during this century. There are also ethical concerns about the intentional destruction of a species, although many would have no ethical qualms about eradicating such a virulent pathogen if doing so were in the best interest of mankind.

# SCOPE

The committee was charged with assessing, from a careful and balanced perspective, the potential scientific and medical information that would be lost were live variola virus no longer available. **The committee was not asked to make a recommendation about destruction or retention of smallpox stocks, and such a determination involves information beyond the purview of the committee.** It is important to recognize that the findings and conclusions about future needs for live variola virus presented in this report fit into a larger, complex policy and ethical debate.

The committee assembled to conduct this assessment has experience with smallpox cases and expertise in viral genetics, molecular biology, immunology, pathogenesis, epidemiology, ethics, antivirals, vaccines, and diagnosis. The committee includes members experienced with poxviruses and a range of other viruses; the chair and two other members observed or treated smallpox patients during field assignments in South Asia. The committee members were selected for their collective ability to provide a broad and balanced perspective on the issues to be addressed.

The committee recognizes that articulation of future scientific needs for live variola virus implies that funds and other resources, including facilities with suitable biological containment provisions, would have to be available to pursue such research. The committee was not, however, able to conduct an assessment of the likelihood of such future support. For this reason, and other reasons discussed more fully in Chapter 12, the committee's findings and conclusions are expressed conditionally: If particular knowledge or capability were to be pursued, would the associated research require live variola virus?

**Moreover, although the committee did not directly address biological warfare as such, it did consider medical and scientific issues that would likely arise if this pathogen were used as a weapon.** We believe the scientific questions likely to be directed to scientists with regard to use of the virus for biological warfare are included in the research-oriented issues encompassed by the committee's charge.

# SCIENTIFIC NEEDS FOR VARIOLA VIRUS

Because scientific research on live variola virus must be conducted in maximum containment facilities, few such efforts have been undertaken in the United States in the past 20 years. There are very few suitable laboratories worldwide, and only two in the United States that would be available for this research. Since smallpox was eradicated, however, understanding of the molecular pathogenesis of viral infections has become considerably more sophisticated. The poxviruses constitute a large, distinctive family of DNA viruses that infect insects, birds, humans, and other mammals. Variola virus is the only uniquely human orthopoxvirus. The only other poxvirus specific to humans is molluscum contagiosum, which causes a rather benign self-limiting skin disease, usually found in children, and does not spread to other parts of the body. Molluscum contagiosum virus is a significant problem only for individuals whose immune systems are compromised. Thus, variola virus interacts with humans in a unique way that cannot be mimicked by other poxviruses. This uniqueness, along with the virus' complex and well-tuned adaptation to the human immune system, suggests a potential for contributing to mankind's knowledge of that system and its defense against infection.

The vertebrate body is an excellent breeding ground for viruses and, by virtue of millions of years of co-evolution, provides conditions that promote virus replication, survival, and transmission. The immune system's response to infecting pathogens is based on a recognition of general molecular patterns in the pathogen or in infected cells. The study of host-virus interactions can illuminate this essential functioning of the immune system [5].

Few would argue the importance of developing new strategies for obtaining knowledge of the human immune system and of mechanisms for modulating human immune responses. More than 50 different viral gene products that modulate the immune system, many from unrelated viruses, have been identified, and it is certain that more will be found. While many of these modulators have similar immune system targets, they show little if any structural similarity [5]. Much remains to be learned from studies of virus-host interactions, and it is likely that those insights could be used to devise better therapies. And because variola virus is human-specific and exhibits unique interactions duplicated by no other known pathogen, studies of variola are likely to provide singular insights.

The variola virus genome is large enough to contain approximately 200 genes, about half of which are devoted to essential functions needed for viral replication and half to interactions with the host. Little is known about how poxviruses enter cells or how cellular receptors interact with the virus. After entry into the cell, virus gene expression, necessary for replication of the viral DNA, begins. Although these processes have not been examined in specific studies using variola virus, they can confidently be predicted because of the extensive similarity between the variola and vaccinia viruses. The genomes of both variola and vaccinia have been sequenced and are 95 percent identical [6].

The genes involved in DNA replication, gene expression, and assembly of new virions are located mainly in the center of the DNA genome. Studies from many laboratories with different strains of poxviruses have shown that the genes involved in virus-host interactions are located near the ends [7, 8]. It is there that most of the differences among the genomes of the poxviruses are found—in those regions determining the interactions with the immune system of the host. Investigations of these interactions are likely to provide fundamental insights into human biology and the functioning of the human immune system. Studies of other viruses provide extensive support for this belief [5]. One notable example is the wholly unexpected finding that proteins within the endoplasmic reticulum can be targeted for destruction and transported into the cytoplasm by virus-encoded gene products [9]. Smallpox was eradicated before the development of many modern techniques of microbiology. As these tools emerged, they were generally applied to studies of pathogens posing current health threats. Partly as a result of the successful eradication of smallpox, therefore, modern analytical techniques have not been applied to enhance understanding of the pathogenesis of variola virus in the human host.

Modern microbiology offers a variety of exploratory tools applicable at different scales, ranging from individual proteins to the entire genome. An assessment of future scientific needs for live variola virus must consider the knowledge that could potentially be derived from the application of these new capabilities, as well as the live variola virus. It also is necessary to consider knowledge that would be greatly facilitated by experiments with variola virus in cell culture, as well as the potential knowledge to be gained from experiments using live variola virus in animal model systems. And given the extensive similarity among the poxvirus genomes, one must consider the extent to which studies with live variola could be supplanted by studies of other poxviruses.

Finally, while the eradication of smallpox was an unequaled public health success, the termination of widespread smallpox vaccination means that virtually the entire global population would now be susceptible should a smallpox outbreak occur. This vulnerability increases the importance of knowledge about variola virus, its pathogenesis, and antiviral strategies that can be employed against it.

## ORGANIZATION OF THIS REPORT

Part II of this report reviews basic knowledge about the pathogen that causes smallpox (Chapter 2), the major features of the disease (Chapter 3), and its spread and strategies for controlling outbreaks (Chapter 4). This part concludes with a brief review of the handling of variola virus stocks following the eradication of smallpox and of research on the virus in the United States (Chapter 5). Part III reviews the scientific needs for variola virus in six areas: the development of antiviral agents (Chapter 6), the development of vaccines (Chapter 7), detection and diagnosis (Chapter 8), bioinformatics (Chapter 9), understanding of the biology of variola virus (Chapter 10), and research on the expressed protein products of variola (Chapter 11). Part IV presents a brief summary and the committee's overall findings and conclusions (Chapter 12). The report ends with a glossary of specialized terms used in the report and brief biographies of the committee members and staff.

# PART II
♦ ♦ ♦ ♦ ♦

# Smallpox and Its Control

# 2

# Variola Virus and Other Orthopoxviruses

Viruses form a distinct group of infectious agents that are fundamentally different from bacteria and protozoa. The infectious particle, called the *virion*, requires the machinery of a host's living cells to reproduce. Viruses become active only after entering a host cell either by membrane fusion (enveloped viruses) or by a process that "uncoats" the virus. The latter process causes the virus to shed some of its outer components so its inner core of genetic material has access to components of the host cell in order to be transcribed and translated. The accepted classification of viruses is based primarily on the morphology of the virion and the nature and structure of the viral nucleic acid. The primary taxonomic division consists of two classes based on nucleic acid content: DNA viruses and RNA viruses. Both categories are further subdivided into viruses that contain either double-stranded or single-stranded DNA or RNA.

The basic taxonomic group is called a *family,* designated by the *"-viridae"* suffix. The family *Poxviridae* contains the largest of all viruses; the virions of the poxviruses are the only virus particles that can be seen with a light microscope. The virions have an ovoid or brick-like shape with dimensions of 400 by 200 nanometers and a linear genome of double-stranded DNA of sufficient length to encode approximately 200 proteins. There are two subfamilies: *Chordopoxvirinae,* which infect vertebrates, and *Entomopoxvirinae,* which infect arthropods. Replication in the cytoplasm of the host cell and the presence of viral enzymes for replication and expression of their genome are characteristic features of all poxviruses. The *Chordipoxvirinae* are divided into subgroups based on morphology, host range, and serological cross-reactivity.

## GENERAL ATTRIBUTES OF ORTHOPOXVIRUSES

The genus Orthopoxvirus is relatively more homogeneous than other members of the *Chordopoxvirinae* subfamily and includes 11 distinct but closely related species showing extensive serological cross-reactivity (see Table 2-1). Neutralization and cross-protection in laboratory animals form the original basis for defining the genus.

The external surface of the poxvirions is ridged in parallel rows that are sometimes arranged helically (see Figure 2-1). As noted, the viral particles contain approximately 200 proteins, about half structural and half nonstructural. Their internal structure is complex. Viewing thin negative-stained sections of virions in an electron microscope reveals that the outer surface is composed of lipid and protein that surrounds the core, which is biconcave (dumbbell-shaped) with two "lateral bodies" of unknown function. The core is composed of tightly compressed nucleoprotein. Poxviruses contain both specific and common proteins. The common proteins induce cross-reactive immunity and account for the ability to vaccinate against disease from another poxvirus of the same genus. There are at least 10 enzymes present in the particle that mediate gene expression. Of all the poxviruses, only those of the genus Orthopoxvirus produce a hemagglutinin antigen (HA).

**TABLE 2-1** Species of the Genus Orthopoxvirus

| Species | Animals Infected | Host Range | Geographic Range |
|---|---|---|---|
| Variola | Human | Narrow | Formerly worldwide |
| Vaccinia | Human,[a] cow, pig, buffalo, rabbit, etc. | Broad | Worldwide[b] |
| Cowpox | Rodent,[a] cow, human, cat, etc. | Broad | Europe |
| Monkeypox | Squirrel,[a] monkey, ape, human | Broad | Western and central Africa |
| Ectromelia | Mouse, mole | Narrow | Europe |
| Camelpox | Camel | Narrow | Africa and Asia |
| Taterapox | Gerbil | Narrow | Western Africa |
| Volepox | Vole | ? | United States |
| Raccoonpox | Raccoon | ? | United States |
| Skunkpox | Skunk | ? | United States |
| Uasin Gishu | Horse | Medium | Eastern Africa |

[a]Primary host.
[b]Secondary to vaccination; no known natural host.

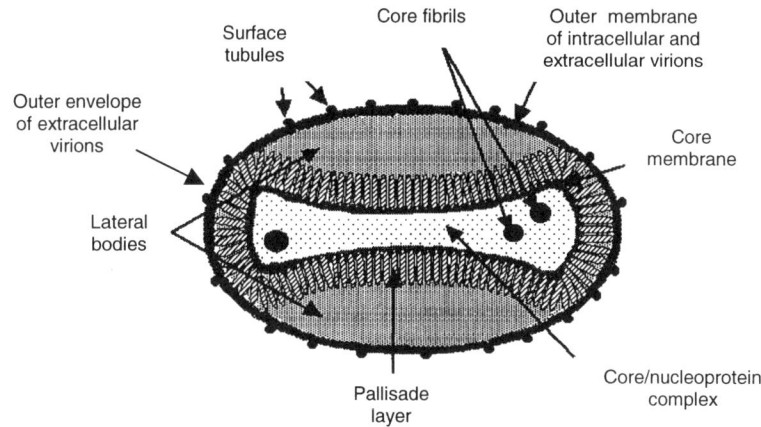

**FIGURE 2-1** Stylized poxvirion from negative stain images [3].

## POXVIRUS REPLICATION

Poxviruses can reproduce only within a host cell. The infection process produces many progeny that are replicas of the parent virus. The first step in the cycle of infection is attachment of the invading virion to the surface of the host cell. Usually the viral DNA genetic material cannot be replicated until it is released from the virion into the host cell.

Most of what is known about poxvirus intracellular growth has come from studies of vaccinia virus. There are two different infectious forms of vaccinia virus—Intracellular Mature Virus (IMV) and Extracellular Enveloped Virus (EEV)—whose virions differ in their role in the virus life cycle, their interaction with the immune system, and the way they bind to and enter cells. However, the question of the relative importance of the IMV and EEV forms for variola virus remains unanswered.

For poxviruses, the synthesis of messenger RNA begins before the genome is uncoated, and is moderated by RNA polymerase and other enzymes packaged within the infectious particle. The *early* messenger RNA is translated into proteins that facilitate the uncoating and replication of the genome and allow transcription of a second class of *intermediate* genes. The intermediate messenger RNA is translated into factors that allow transcription of the *late* class of genes. The late messenger RNA is translated into the structural and enzyme components of the virion. The newly replicated progeny genomes are incorporated into the virions being assembled. In culture, the last step of the growth cycle is the exit of progeny virions by eventual lysis or less frequently by exocytosis, in which virions are enveloped by virus-altered cell membranes of the host cell. The progeny virions can then spread the infection to neighboring cells, to other sites, or to other individuals [1, 10]. Viremia in vivo is largely cell-associated, and mechanisms of spread are not fully understood.

Within several hours of infection, so-called "toxic," or cytopathic, changes occur in infected cells. This process involves general shutdown of the synthesis of host DNA, RNA, and protein, as well as changes in the cell architecture. These changes occur as the virus takes over the metabolic machinery of the cell for its own purposes.

## PROPERTIES OF SPECIFIC ORTHOPOXVIRUSES

Poxviruses contain large double-stranded genomes and differ from most other DNA viruses in that they replicate in the cytoplasm rather than in the nucleus of susceptible cells. Selected properties of five orthopoxvirus species are described here because of the relevance of these species to the assessment of future scientific needs for live variola virus.*

**Variola Virus.** Variola is a human-specific virus. Generally it can be readily distinguished from other orthopoxviruses capable of infecting man (vaccinia, cowpox, monkeypox) by the characteristic small white pocks produced on the chorioallantoic membrane of developing 12- to 15-day-old chick embryos and the ceiling temperature of growth.

How, where, or when variola virus originated is not known. The basic question regarding the origin of a human-specific virus is how long ago, in terms of biological evolution, the viral species in question developed the capacity to be maintained indefinitely through human-to-human spread. Indefinite maintenance of a virus in populations of various sizes depends on three factors: (1) certain characteristics of the virus, notably its capacity to undergo antigenic change; (2) characteristics of the pathogenesis of the infection, especially the quality of the immune response and whether persistent infection or recurrence of infectivity occurs; and (3) characteristics of the population biology of the host, notably the rate of accession of new susceptible subjects. It has been estimated that a population of about 200,000 susceptible individuals would be necessary to support a sustained infection with humans as the sole host, and that this circumstance could have occurred only after the introduction of irrigated agriculture, about 10,000 years ago, had engendered the first great population explosion.

Two possibilities could explain the existence of a human-specific virus that has been recognized for 2,000 to 3,000 years. First, humans could have acquired the virus from some animal host in which the virus could be maintained in

---

* Much of the discussion in this section and in Chapters 2 and 3 based on *Smallpox and Its Eradication,* Fenner et al. (1988).

larger numbers and had a much shorter generation time than in humans. Second, humans (or perhaps protohumans) may long have been the host of an ancestral "variola virus" that produced a different sort of disease that could persist in small groups of hunter-gatherers. The first of these possibilities appears probable. While monkeypox is a likely candidate since it causes a disease in humans that is very similar to smallpox, the variola virus genome exhibits greater similarity to other orthopoxviruses.

From the time it was first recognized until the end of the 19th century, smallpox was regarded as a uniformly severe disease with case-fatality rates in unvaccinated individuals of up to 40 percent. As noted in Chapter 1, in about 1900 a milder form of smallpox was identified with case-fatality rates of 1 percent or less. This milder form of smallpox is called *variola minor,* while the term *variola major* refers to the classical, more serious form. A more detailed description of the pathogenesis of and immune response to variola virus infections is presented in Chapter 3.

**Vaccinia Virus.** Vaccinia virus has been propagated by humans for use as a smallpox vaccine for the past 200 years. There are no known natural hosts of vaccinia virus, and its origin is obscure. All present strains of vaccinia virus are genetically related, although they exhibit different biological properties in the laboratory. Most strains have a wide host range in experimental animals, and all exhibit rapid growth on the chorioallantoic membrane cultures. Since the early 1980s, strains of vaccinia have been engineered to express genetic information for other viral and bacterial antigens or immunomodulatory proteins. Vaccination against smallpox is most effective by infection of the skin with vaccinia virus, followed by extension of replication to the lymph nodes and spleen, which elicits cell-mediated and humoral immune responses that provide protection against infection with variola virus.

The clinical events following primary inoculation of the skin with vaccinia virus are more rapid than the course of a natural smallpox infection, and are localized rather than generalized. Inoculation produces a papule at the vaccination site on the third day after vaccination. This papule becomes vesicular within 2 or 3 days. As with smallpox, the vesicle soon becomes pustular, mostly as a result of the entry of polymorphonuclear cells, the influx of which is induced by the viral infection. The surrounding skin becomes much more tender than in smallpox, and the lesions reach maximum size between 8 and 12 days after infection. At this time the lymph nodes are more or less enlarged and tender, and the subject sometimes experiences mild fever and malaise. The pustule dries from the center outward to become a scab that falls off about 3 weeks after vaccination to leave a typical pitted scar.

**Monkeypox Virus.** Human monkeypox is a systemic disease with a generalized pustular rash that is usually clinically indistinguishable from that of smallpox. Monkeypox virus was discovered in 1958 when it was isolated from the lesions of captive monkeys at the State Serum Institute in Copenhagen. Monkeypox virus has a broad host range that includes most common laboratory animals. Monkeypox antibodies have been found in various wild animals, especially squirrels in Zaire.

The first case of human monkeypox was identified in Zaire in 1970, followed by four cases in Liberia and one in Sierra Leone. Clinically, human monkeypox closely resembles ordinary smallpox. The most obvious clinical difference is a pronounced lymph-node enlargement with monkeypox, which typically occurs in the neck and groin, but can be more generalized. Swollen lymph glands and fever precede the rash in most cases.

Prospective studies in Zaire between 1981 and 1986 have indicated that three-fourths of human monkeypox infections are attributable to direct contact with animals; the remainder can be traced to contact with infected persons. Whereas the person-to-person transmission rate to unvaccinated individuals in close contact ranges up to 70 percent for smallpox, it is about 8 percent for monkeypox. Serial transmission of monkeypox involving more than two or three people is rare. While monkeypox probably has existed in the tropical rain forests of Africa for a long time, it apparently has never established a continuous person-to-person infection in a human population. Preliminary results from sequencing of DNA fragments of monkeypox virus isolates obtained at various times since 1970 suggest that the virus has changed very little during this period. At present, there is no clear evidence that the rate of human-to-human transmission of monkeypox is likely to increase.[*]

**Cowpox Virus.** Cowpox is of interest primarily because of its role in the discovery of vaccination. The occurrence of a sporadic pox disease in cows that is transmissible to humans had been known for centuries when Edward Jenner, an English country physician, brought it to public attention (see the discussion of "Immunity Against Smallpox" in Chapter 3). The virus can infect a variety of animals, and is probably maintained over time in rodents. Its genome is the largest of all the orthopoxviruses, and deletion mutations occur commonly, producing progeny with smaller genomes. None of the strains of cowpox virus that have been examined looks at all like that of variola virus.

**Mousepox (Infectious Ectromelia) Virus.** This virus, discovered in 1930, is a natural pathogen of mice, causing serious disease with a rash in outbred and several inbred strains. It has been used to study the molecular basis of the virulence of orthopoxviruses since it has the advantage that the mouse, by far the best experimental animal for such studies, is its natural host [11]. Mousepox,

---

[*] Joseph J. Esposito, Personal communication, December 1998.

however, is not fully comparable to variola virus because the route of infection is usually skin abrasion rather than inhalation, and ectromelia is unique among the orthopoxviruses in that the spleen and liver are major target organs for viral replication.

# 3

# Clinical Features of Smallpox

The term *pathogenesis* is used to describe the mechanisms involved in the production of disease, from the spread of infection through the body to the molecular and physiological responses of host cells to a pathogen. *Immune response* is the constellation of mechanisms by which the host limits continued multiplication of the pathogen. These mechanisms include T cell and B cell responses that are specific for the organism and are acquired during the course of the infection. Some of these mechanisms are *innate,* while others are *adaptive.*

The pathogenesis of smallpox has been studied in three ways: (1) by using material from human patients; (2) by conducting experiments with variola virus infection of nonhuman primates; and (3) by conducting experiments with model infections in mice, rabbits, and monkeys using related orthopoxviruses. Investigations in human subjects prior to eradication were limited to virological and serological tests of hospitalized smallpox patients or case contacts and case histories. Much of our understanding of the pathogenesis of generalized orthopoxvirus infections is based on studies carried out with ectromelia (mousepox).

## ENTRY AND INFECTION

The usual entry of variola virus is through the respiratory tract with infection of the oropharyngeal (mouth) or respiratory (trachea and lung) mucosa. Secretions from the mouth and nose, rather than scab material, are the most important source of human-to-human transmission. The initial infection in the oropharynx or respiratory tract produces neither symptoms nor local lesions, and patients are not infectious until an oropharyngeal enanthem appears at the end of the primary incubation period. Transmission to others is generally through coughing out of virions in oropharyngeal secretions. Patients are most infectious during the first week of rash. Scab material forms as the rash dries and usually consists of large fragments of cellular debris, with virions bound within a dense, fibrous mesh containing a large amount of the antiviral substance interferon. Infectious virus is difficult to release from scabs except by mechanical grinding.

*Inoculation smallpox* sometimes occurs when variola virus is introduced into the skin either intentionally or accidentally. A local skin lesion appears on the third or fourth day, with fever and constitutional symptoms beginning on the eighth day. The incubation period is typically 2 to 3 days shorter than in natural smallpox. The rash, which is usually less severe than in naturally acquired smallpox, appears on the tenth or eleventh day. The milder course of disease stemming from deliberate variola inoculation was the basis for variolation, which preceded Jenner's use of cowpox and the subsequent use of vaccinia inoculation as a preventive for smallpox (as discussed further below).

Very rarely, vaccinia vaccination produces *dissemination vaccinia,* a systemic infection characterized by malaise combined with a generalized rash similar to inoculation lesions. In another condition, called *progressive vaccinia,* the inoculation lesion fails to heal, and secondary lesions sometimes appear elsewhere. Both conditions are problematic predominantly for individuals with deficient immune mechanisms.

Variola major caused severe problems in pregnant women. Abortions and stillbirths were frequent, and a majority of the babies born to infected women in hospital died within 15 days, most within 3 days. About half of the babies acquired infection in utero or at the time of delivery.

## DISSEMINATION

The appearance of high fever and then lesions on the skin marks the end of the incubation period. Smallpox pathogenesis is a poorly understood series of events in which the virus first disseminates locally, then through the lymphatic system, and finally to the skin without affecting vital organs. In mousepox, the primary source of molecular studies of orthopoxvirus pathogenesis, the infection moves from the respiratory tract to the liver and spleen following breach of the macrophage barrier. The virus then replicates extensively in both organs, which produces semiconfluent necrosis. About a day after infection of the liver and spleen, large numbers of virions are liberated into the bloodstream, leading to secondary infection of the skin, kidneys, lungs, intestines, and other organs. This phase is followed by an interval of 2 or 3 days during which the virus replicates and reaches a high titer before visible changes are apparent in the infected organs.

As noted earlier, mousepox is unusual among the generalized orthopoxvirus infections in that the spleen and liver are the major target organs for viral replication. There is inadequate evidence regarding exactly where the virus replicates during a smallpox infection. The likely sites for viral replication are the lymphoid organs (spleen, bone marrow, lymph nodes), but extensive necrosis does not occur in those sites. At this stage, the virus in the blood is largely cell-associated.

## THE RASH

The primary event that triggers the production of focal lesions in orthopoxvirus infections is the localization of virus particles in the small dermal blood vessels. Subsequently, adjacent epidermal cells are infected, and skin lesions develop. The earliest change is dilation of the capillaries in the papillary layer of the dermis, followed by swelling of the endothelial cells in the walls of these vessels and subsequently perivascular cuffing with lymphocytes, plasma cells, and macrophages. Following these early changes, the cells of the Malpighian layer become swollen and vacuolated. The cells continue to increase in size, and the nucleus usually disappears or is lysed. The cell membrane then ruptures, and the vacuoles coalesce to produce the early vesicle. Because this coalescence occurs quickly, a true papule is rarely seen, and the lesions appear vesicular almost from the beginning. Except on the palms and soles, umbilication is a common feature of skin lesions in smallpox. It is due mainly to swelling of the cells around the vesicle and proliferation of the basal cells surrounding the lesion, so that the periphery of the vesicle is raised above its center. The mechanisms that allow the localization of variola virus in the skin and the characteristic "centrifugal" distribution of the rash are not known.

With the development of an effective immune response (described below), healing begins. The contents of the pustule become desiccated, and reestablishment of the epithelial skin layer occurs between the cavity of the pustule and the underlying dermis. The pustule contents become a crusty scab. On the soles and palms, the horny layer of the skin is very thick, and the dried exudate often remains for a long period if not removed artificially.

The face bears the heaviest crop of lesions in most cases of smallpox, and scarring is more common there than elsewhere. Although cells of other skin appendages (hair follicles and sweat glands) are relatively unaffected by variola virus, cells of the sebaceous glands are highly susceptible. Degeneration occurs simultaneously in several parts of the gland, leading to extensive necrosis. When healing occurs, the defect in the dermis fills with granulation tissue, which frequently shrinks, leaving localized facial pockmarks.

## LESIONS OF THE MUCOUS MEMBRANES

Although the oropharynx and respiratory tract are usually regarded as the portal of entry for smallpox, primary lesions have not been observed in these areas. The mucous membranes in which enanthem lesions later develop are, in order of frequency, the pharynx and uvula, the larynx, the tongue, and the upper part of the trachea and esophagus. Lesions of the lower trachea and bronchi are much less frequent.

Epithelial cells in mucous membranes are not as tightly packed as in skin, and there is no horny layer. Therefore, there is more pronounced exudation of fluid into the subepithelial tissues than occurs with dermal lesions. This exudation and the subsequent separation of cells and their degeneration are the earliest changes. Instead of a vesicle, the extensive necrosis in the epithelial cells, unrestrained by a horny layer, leads to ulceration. Later, increasing vascularization takes on the appearance of granulation tissue, with numerous polymorphonuclear leukocytes in the demarcation zone beneath the necrotic epithelium.

The lack of a horny, keratinized cell layer permits the lesions on the mucous membranes to ulcerate soon after their formation, releasing large amounts of highly infectious virus into the saliva. Viral titers, or amounts of virus in throat swabs, are at their maximum on the third and fourth days of the disease. In fatal cases, virus is usually still present in throat swabs at the time of death. The onset of infectivity coincides with the development of the rash and is due to the release of the virus from the ulcerated surfaces of these skin and mucosal lesions.

## EFFECTS ON OTHER ORGANS

Death is usually the result of disseminated intravascular coagulation, hypotension, and cardiovascular collapse; these are exacerbated by clotting defects in the rare hemorrhagic type of smallpox. The endothelial cells lining the sinusoids of the liver are often swollen and occasionally proliferating or necrotic. Reticulum cell hyperplasia occurs in the bone marrow and spleen. The spleen is usually engorged and contains many large lymphoid cells. The liver is generally considerably heavier than normal, but this does not appear to be due to engorgement or fatty infiltration. Encephalitis is an occasional complication.

## IMMUNE RESPONSE

The human immune response to viruses is a complicated process about which much has yet to be discovered. Furthermore, knowledge of interactions between the immune system and variola virus is limited because modern techniques for the study of immune responses were developed after smallpox was eradicated.

At least three types of cells are involved: macrophages, dendritic cells, and lymphocytes. Macrophages and dendritic cells process antigens for presentation to T cells (thymus-derived lymphocytes, of which there are several subclasses). Macrophages and dendritic cells may acquire antigen at a given location from which they migrate to specialized lymphoid tissue—lymph nodes—the architecture of which allows for the cell-cell interactions required for a proper immune response. Importantly, certain antigen-presenting cells are able to be infected with different viruses, including orthopoxviruses.

B cells are responsible for producing immunoglobulin, and often require help from T cells to do so. Such B lymphocytes have immunoglobulins on their cell surface that function as antigen-specific receptors. When an antigen triggers the B cell receptor and when appropriate help is delivered to the B cells by T lymphocytes or their secreted products, the B cells are stimulated to respond clonally. B cells differentiate into antibody-secreting plasma cells or long-lived memory cells, which are critically important in mounting a secondary response upon re-exposure to antigen.

While immunoglobulins can recognize antigen directly, the antigen-specific receptors on T lymphocytes interact with antigens on the surface of cells that present antigen in the form of short peptides (8–15 amino acids) in a complex with products of the Major Histocompatibility Complex (MHC). The generation of the peptides requires the proteolytic conversion of protein antigens into suitably sized peptides (antigen processing). The complicated series of reactions between antigen-presenting and T cells serves to announce to the immune system the presence of intracellular pathogens such as viruses. Not surprisingly, a number of viruses have evolved mechanisms that deflect this process, presumably helping them avoid immune recognition.

T cells respond specifically to MHC antigen presentation by clonal expansion. When activated, they secrete active substances called cytokines. As with B cells, a subset of activated T cells become long-lived memory cells. There are subclasses of T cells that have different functions. Some act to modulate B cells and other T cells by enhancing or suppressing their proliferation or their production of antibodies or cytokines. T cells that recognize viral proteins differentiate on contact with a specific antigen to release cytokines, such as gamma-interferon. Such cells cause delayed-type hypersensitivity reactions, thereby attracting other inflammatory cells to the sites of infection. Certain T cells are cytotoxic and actively destroy cells exhibiting specific viral proteins composed of MHC products on their surface.

During infection with a virus as complex as an orthopoxvirus, antibodies specific to many different viral proteins are generated. Antibodies of three types have received specific attention: (1) those that neutralize viral infectivity; (2) those that, in conjunction with other proteins, lead to lysis of virus-infected cells; and (3) those that combine with circulating antigens to produce immune complexes. Information about T cell responses to smallpox is very limited. However, in other viral infections, T cell responses often precede the appearance of neutralizing or other antibodies. Clearance of virus in many situations correlates with activation and expansion of virus-specific T cells. The kinetics of the appearance of antibodies is often slower than the initiation of T cell responses in the generation of cytotoxic T cells and T cells that produce interferon-gamma or other cytokines. This may be the case for smallpox as well, although the molecular tools needed to evaluate this question were not available when the disease was prevalent.

In nonhemorrhagic smallpox, hemagglutinin-inhibiting (HI) and neutralizing antibody titers increase from about the sixth day of illness (approximately 18 days after infection), and most patients develop immunoprecipitating antibodies that can be demonstrated by Ouchterlony-like gel precipitation assay about 2 days later. Patients with the rare hemorrhagic type of smallpox have much-reduced neutralizing antibody responses. HI titers rise and are approximately the same for patients with either ordinary or hemorrhagic smallpox.

Lowered numbers of both T cells and B cells have been observed in smallpox patients, but the subtypes of the T cells have not been determined.

The best information on the relative importance of cell-mediated and humoral immune responses to orthopoxvirus infections in humans comes from studies of human subjects in immune-deficient states who are subsequently vaccinated with vaccinia virus. In children with immunological defects in cell-mediated immunity, vaccinia virus replicates without restriction, resulting in a continually progressive primary lesion, persistent viremia, and widespread secondary viral infection of many organs. In patients with thymic dysplasia and partially or completely intact immunoglobulin-synthesizing capacity (Nezelof's syndrome), the progression is slower and less persistent, but usually results in death. Delayed-type hypersensitivity reactions are not evoked in patients with progressive vaccinia, nor can their peripheral blood lymphocytes be stimulated to undergo mitosis by exposure to inactivated vaccinia virus. Although neutralizing antibody is sometimes present in the serum, its presence does not prevent the development of progressive vaccinia if cell-mediated immunity is defective.

Orthopoxvirus-specific T cell and B cell memory can be thought of as involving previously induced lymphocytes that persist as long-lived but nonactivated cells sequestered in lymphoid tissue and in the recirculating pool of lymphocytes. The effectiveness of memory T cells in providing protective immunity against orthopoxviruses decreases as the interval between primary and secondary infection increases.

## IMMUNITY AGAINST SMALLPOX

All orthopoxviruses induce cross-protective immunity in susceptible laboratory animals. Indeed, that is one of the ways of identifying members of the genus and is the basis for currently available vaccines. Among the orthopoxviruses that infect humans, cowpox and vaccinia viruses usually produce only local lesions and minimal systemic disturbance. Variola and monkeypox viruses cause serious systemic disturbance with high case-fatality rates. The observation that recurrences of smallpox were very rare had been made in ancient times, and led to attempts to ameliorate the severity of smallpox by administering pustular fluid or dried scab material to the nostrils or skin of persons who had not yet contracted smallpox. Much later, it was observed that similar protection against smallpox could be obtained by administering cowpox or vaccinia virus.

The process of inoculating smallpox material is called *variolation* to distinguish it from vaccination, which uses cowpox or vaccinia virus. After variolation of the skin, a primary lesion develops at the inoculation site on about the third day, and satellite pustules are common. But the rash is usually much less severe than with naturally occurring smallpox. Historically, case-fatality rates were between 0.5 and 2 percent after variolation, compared with 20 to 30 percent from natural smallpox. Since the virus material used was not attenuated, it was possible for those receiving variolation to transmit ordinary smallpox to susceptible contacts.

Early in the 18th century, the variolation procedure spread through the Balkans into central Europe and from Turkey to Great Britain and the rest of Europe. Subsequently, Jenner confirmed earlier observations that a person who had suffered cowpox did not get smallpox. In 1796 he took matter from cowpox lesions on the hand of Sarah Nelmes, a young dairymaid, and used it to inoculate an 8-year-old boy. After the boy's slight fever and low-grade lesion disappeared, Jenner attempted to variolate him by inoculating him with smallpox. The primary lesion did not develop, and protection was complete [12]. The educated public was receptive to this discovery. Jenner's vaccine was a way of providing the advantages of variolation without the associated risks, and there was no doubt that cowpox produced a much less severe disease than variolation. To recognize Jenner's contribution, Louis Pasteur later proposed that this method of protecting against infectious diseases be called *vaccination* and the product used a *vaccine,* although the general process is now usually called *immunization.*

At some unknown point in time, vaccinia virus became substituted for cowpox virus, probably because it produced generally milder lesions and lower fever. Modern vaccination against smallpox consists of abrading the skin with vaccinia virus, which may subsequently spread to the lymph nodes and spleen, organs heavily involved in initiating the immune response (as discussed earlier). The result of spread to these sites is the induction of cell-mediated and humoral immunity, and long-lived memory T and B cells that recognize the virus. Replication of variola virus is completely prevented for a few years, and thereafter replication is limited so that infection is subclinical, causing no symptoms. Immunity wanes over time and can decline to levels that do not protect against illness, although the severity of disease is likely to be reduced.

Passive immunization, as a natural consequence of either transmission of antibodies from mother to progeny or the administration of antisera, is less effective in modifying the course of disease than active immunization involving live virus. Active immunity, whether elicited by vaccination or the disease, provokes the complete range of cell-mediated and humoral immune responses, whereas passive immunization provides only the antibodies present in the source of the sera.

Three groups of complications occurred in a small number of vaccinated subjects: abnormal skin eruptions, disorders affecting the central nervous system, and a variety of other rarer or less severe complications. Although trivial compared with the problems historically associated with smallpox, these complications posed significant health risks when smallpox receded. Therefore, vaccination was discontinued once smallpox had been eradicated globally.

# 4

# Epidemiology

The earliest writers on smallpox—Ko Hung in China, Vagbhata in India, and al-Razi in Asia Minor—describe it primarily as a disease of children. This is a mark of well-established endemic prevalence, and argues that smallpox had been present in those areas for centuries. At the beginning of the 20th century—a hundred years after the introduction of vaccination—smallpox was endemic in almost every country of the world. In 1920, the only countries with large enough populations to support endemic smallpox where it was absent were Australia and New Zealand, which were protected by distance and effective seaport quarantines. A population with at least 200,000 susceptible individuals is required to support endemic smallpox.

## CHARACTERISTICS OF HISTORICAL OUTBREAKS

All histories of smallpox record periods punctuated by major epidemics, which can be distinguished by two epidemiologically distinct situations. The first was when smallpox was introduced into a location where it had not occurred previously, or at least not for many years, so that a large portion of the population was susceptible. This led to epidemics affecting all age groups and producing considerable social disruption since most breadwinners were afflicted. The second situation was one in which, for a variety of demographic, climatic, and other reasons, optimum conditions for transmission fluctuated so that epidemics occurred every few years against a background of endemicity. This situation was much less socially disruptive than the first because there were always many smallpox-immune adults.

The size and density of the population at risk affect the chances of contact between susceptible and infectious persons, and thus the rapidity with which smallpox spreads. While very brief exposures of susceptible persons could occasionally lead to infection, epidemiologists engaged in the global smallpox eradication program concluded that the disease spreads rather slowly. Because of the importance of face-to-face contact, the household constituted by far the most frequently affected group. However, hospitals, schools, and public events also contributed significantly to the spread of smallpox. Because of the long incubation period of the infection (see Chapter 3), infected travelers could cover long distances while apparently healthy and could thus introduce smallpox into areas far removed from the source of their infection. In the past, fellow travelers were sometimes infected when ambulant patients, probably infected with vaccine-modified smallpox, traveled in close contact with others. If an outbreak were to occur today, however, most infected travelers would become infectious after arriving at their destinations, some of which would likely be far from their point of infection.

Subclinical infections with variola virus seldom occurred, except when individuals who had been vaccinated were in close contact with infectious cases. These individuals rarely transmitted smallpox to others and were of little epidemiological importance. An attack of smallpox is followed by death or recovery. Persistent, latent, or recurrent infection does not occur, and cases are not infectious after the rash disappears. Survivors generally have immunity for life. Smallpox spread slowly, with an interval of 2 to 3 weeks between each generation of cases. Even during winter and spring, when smallpox appeared to be more easily transmitted, an infectious patient seldom infected as many as five other persons.

## LIKELY CHARACTERISTICS OF FUTURE SMALLPOX OUTBREAKS

Only three smallpox outbreaks that occurred during and following the eradication program were clearly identified as attributable to accidents at laboratories handling live variola virus. Regulations governing the handling of live variola virus and related clinical material subsequently became much more stringent, so the most likely source of a future outbreak would be deliberate release by terrorists or rogue nations.

In an accidental release, those infected could range from a single individual to a moderate number of individuals. Deliberate release, however, would probably result in essentially simultaneous infection of many individuals. If the release exposed persons who were highly mobile, the relatively lengthy incubation period of the infection could enable the infection to spread widely before being identified. Thereafter the outbreak would probably resemble those that occurred historically in places where smallpox was not endemic and that came to light only after the infection had been passed to the second generation of patients [13].

Individuals infected with variola virus become sick before they are fully infectious to others. For this reason, the spread of smallpox historically in nonendemic areas was principally to close family members, even when a high proportion of the population had not been vaccinated [13, 14]. Although the human-to-human transmission rate of the disease can be high, an individual infected patient did not have numerous close contacts unless he or she was in a large household, a hospital, or some other institution (homes for elderly, for example, suffered in recorded outbreaks). This experience suggests that a future outbreak of smallpox would infect people of all ages, but that the epidemic would not become explosive, as would be the case with a disease transmitted prior to the onset of illness.

## CONTROL STRATEGIES

Herd immunity (a large number of immune individuals in the exposed population) limits the spread of diseases transmitted by subclinically infected persons or patients who are fully mobile. It is less important for smallpox, since once infectious, patients are typically confined to bed. Hindsight reveals that the vast majority of vaccinations during the panics associated with smallpox outbreaks in the past were unnecessary since transmission was limited mainly to close contacts within the household or hospital. Prompt diagnosis, isolation, and vaccination of close contacts is of much greater importance. This was essentially the strategy employed in the global eradication program.

Given that the disease would probably be transmitted to the second generation of patients before being diagnosed, however, suitable antiviral therapies would be of great value. Yet, as discussed in Chapter 6, no currently available antiviral agent is effective against variola virus infection, development of such an agent would be time-consuming and costly, and its therapeutic effectiveness would remain unproven until an outbreak occurred.

A smallpox outbreak would be a medical emergency. Criteria for contraindications to vaccination and for the type of vaccine to be used would need to be less strict than in the absence of the disease. Rapidity of response would probably be of greater immediate concern than safety. Nevertheless, the considerable number of individuals immunocompromised as a result of the AIDS epidemic and increased organ transplant and chemotherapy procedures constitute a special risk since inoculating these individuals with the traditional live vaccinia vaccine is not acceptable (see also Chapter 7).

The lessons of the past can help us prepare for future smallpox outbreaks. At the same time, however, the techniques of the past need to be augmented by the best contemporary knowledge available.

# 5

# Variola Virus Stocks Following Eradication of Smallpox

The World Health Organization (WHO) Intensified Smallpox Eradication Program was established in 1967. It included a global surveillance program, isolation of smallpox patients, and vaccination of the possible contacts of patients. Eradication of smallpox constitutes one of the greatest successes of modern medicine. After the World Health Assembly sanctioned the WHO declaration of 1980 that smallpox had been eradicated, WHO established a Committee on Orthopoxvirus Infections (COI) to advise on steps to be taken in the posteradication era and to monitor the conduct of those steps [15]. COI has continued to meet about every 4 years since that time. The question of whether smallpox virus should be retained and the conditions for its retention are among the most important issues faced by COI. The issue has been brought to formal vote at several COI meetings, usually with the majority favoring destruction.

Throughout its deliberations, COI has faced two strongly held, conflicting points of view [15]. Some scientists and many countries, especially those that experienced endemic smallpox most recently, greatly fear the reintroduction of smallpox and have argued passionately for taking all available measures to avert this possibility, including early destruction of all known stocks of the virus. It is recognized that this measure would provide no absolute guarantee against the possibility that some stocks of virus unknown to WHO might continue to exist. COI has also acknowledged that there is great scientific value in the stocks, but has expressed the belief that the risk of keeping the virus outweighs the potential benefits. It is generally believed that an international agreement to destroy the virus stocks would diminish the likelihood of the virus being released. On the other side, some scientists have argued for retention of the known stocks, expressing concerns about losing experimental material that could provide important information regarding viral pathogenesis in humans, as well as about establishing a precedent for the deliberate destruction of an archived species and the associated loss of genetic information. These concerns are implicitly seen as outweighing the risks of keeping the virus. Many participants in the COI discussions have found themselves in broad agreement in perceiving merit in both points of view. Efforts to reconcile the two incompatible policy stances have been a continuing challenge for COI and others.

## ESTABLISHMENT OF INTERNATIONAL REPOSITORIES

Starting in 1977, the number of laboratories known to be holding stocks of variola virus was reduced until by the end of 1983 all known stocks were held in only two WHO Collaborating Centres—the U.S. Centers for Disease Control and Prevention (CDC) in Atlanta, Georgia, and the Research Institute for Viral Pre-parations in Moscow, Russia [1]. The Russian stocks were transferred in 1994 to the State Center of Virology and Biotechnology (VECTOR) in Kotsovo, Russia, which subsequently became the WHO Collaborating Centre for Orthopoxvirus Diagnostics.

Use of these remaining variola stocks at CDC and VECTOR is restricted to approved Biological Safety Level 4 (BSL-4) conditions (see Box 5-1). WHO periodically conducts safety and security inspections of the facilities. Inventories of the samples at each institution are on file at WHO. COI recommended that cloned fragment libraries of selected strains be prepared and that selected prototypical strains be sequenced [15].

In addition, handling of cloned DNA fragments of the variola virus genome follows the recommendations issued in a 1994 COI report [16]:

- The two international repositories for storage, maintenance, and distribution of cloned DNA fragments of variola virus are CDC and VECTOR.
- Each sample is identified by nucleotide sequence determination.
- A register of cloned material is maintained, containing full descriptive and sequence information.
- Clones are distributed to research laboratories requesting them if:

    – The clones will not be further distributed to third parties.
    – The clones are not to be used for insertion of variola DNA into vaccinia virus or related poxviruses. No laboratory other than the international repositories is permitted to hold clones representing more than 20 percent of the variola virus genome at any one time.

> **BOX 5-1 Laboratory Safety**
>
> Because of its extreme virulence, variola virus must be handled in maximum containment facilities (BSL-4). These facilities consist of a separate building or clearly isolated section of a building with a sealed internal shell. Outer and inner change rooms separated by a shower are provided for personnel entering and exiting the facility. A double-doored autoclave, fumigation chamber, or ventilated airlock is provided for passage of materials not brought into the facility through the change room. Sewer and ventilation lines contain high-efficiency particulate air (HEPA) filters. Special individual supply and exhaust air ventilation is provided for laboratory workers, and pressure differentials are maintained to ensure the inward flow of air toward areas where the potential for hazard is highest [17].
>
> There have been only two maximum containment facilities in the United States: one at CDC and one at Fort Detrick, in Frederick, Maryland. Recently a BSL-4 laboratory dedicated to the study of tuberculosis was opened at the National Institutes of Health. Since these limited facilities have generally been devoted to the study of pathogens perceived to pose a more immediate threat than smallpox, there has been very little research on variola. The scarcity of laboratory facilities suitable and authorized for studying live variola virus is a serious constraint on the U.S. capability to undertake the research discussed in this report.
>
> It would be possible to alter the variola virus genome to remove its capability for surviving outside the laboratory. For example, the uracil DNA glycosylase (UDG) gene could be knocked out, so that the virus could grow only in cells that expressed the viral UDG [18]. Currently, this approach would be limited to cell tissue studies, but it could, with a change in the regulations to recognize the inability of the altered virus to survive, enable use of the much more common BSL-3 facilities that utilize safety cabinets and other personal protective or physical containment devices [17]. Present regulations, however, require that no material handled in BSL-4 facilities can be opened at lower containment unless it is killed by means such as autoclaving, irradiating, or chemical treatment.

Analysis performed mainly at CDC and VECTOR has produced about 750,000 bases of variola virus genome DNA sequence. The complete genome of variola major virus Bangladesh-1975 (GenBank #L22579) has been sequenced. With the exception of small regions at the ends of the DNA, the variola major virus India-1967 (GenBank X69198) and the variola minor alastrim virus Brazil/Garcia-1966 (EMBL Y167080) have also been fully sequenced.*

---

* Joseph J. Esposito, Personal communication, December 1998.

The collections of variola virus samples held at CDC (approximately 450 samples, including CDC isolates and isolates deposited by the U.S. Army, the American Type Culture Collection, the National Health Institute of Japan, the National Health Institute of the Netherlands, and the United Kingdom Microbiological Research Establishment) and at VECTOR (120 samples comprising Moscow Institute of Viral Preparations isolates from about 20 countries) comprise isolates from clinical samples and material used in variolation that was collected from 1950 through the 1970s. The samples at CDC and VECTOR are preserved as frozen material (generally early passage material) from cell cultures or avian chorioallantoic membranes infected with lesion material; a portion of the samples is lyophilized. Approximately 27 samples at CDC and 17 at VECTOR comprise original lesion material from smallpox patients. Generally, the source of each isolate is documented, but the extent of that documentation varies. The samples, some of which are duplicated, do not represent a complete archive of taxonomically characterized strains from the different outbreaks in recent history.[*]

## DECISION BY THE WORLD HEALTH ASSEMBLY TO DESTROY VARIOLA VIRUS STOCKS

In 1986 and again in 1990, COI affirmed the desirability of destroying variola virus stocks and intact DNA (but not cloned DNA fragments) after satisfactory progress had been made with sequencing, mapping, and cloning [15]. COI subsequently decided that before making a final decision with regard to destruction of the virus, it would consult more widely with the scientific community [15]. In 1993, a special roundtable discussion took place in Glasgow at the International Congress on Virology. Alternative views regarding destruction of the virus were published in companion articles in *Science,* and the views of a number of professional bodies were solicited, several of which formally endorsed destruction.

After a 1994 review of the issues and progress made in mapping, cloning, and sequencing of strains, COI voted unanimously to recommend that the virus be destroyed. All but two members recommended June 1996 as a target date, the others calling for a delay until June 1999. COI recommended to the Executive Board of the World Health Assembly that a resolution calling for the destruction of all known stocks of variola virus in June 1996 be endorsed and forwarded for action to the World Health Assembly.

At the ensuing WHO Executive Board meeting, the United States supported the decision to destroy the virus at the end of June 1996. However, as a result of further discussion and debate at that meeting and at the subsequent meeting of the World Health Assembly, the decision was made to defer destruction of the

---

[*] Joseph J. Esposito, Personal communication, December 1998.

remaining stocks of variola virus, intact viral genomic DNA, and clinical specimens or other material containing live variola virus until June 1999, and then only after a reaffirmation of the decision at the May 1999 World Health Assembly meeting [19].

At the most recent COI meeting in January 1999, the committee voted in favor of the destruction of the remaining stocks still kept at the WHO Collaborating Centres in the Russian Federation and the United States. The vote, however, was not unanimous. Five of the nine committee members voted for immediate destruction, two voted for eventual destruction following a review in 5 years, and two supported indefinite retention of the stocks [20].

## U.S. RESEARCH ON SMALLPOX

In 1995, continuing disagreements within the U.S. government as to the appropriate policy on destruction of variola virus stocks led to the appointment of civilian advisers to the U.S. Department of Health and Human Services (DHHS) and the U.S. Department of Defense (DOD) to reexamine the issues involved. These advisors represented the Board of Scientific Counselors of the National Center for Infectious Diseases at CDC and the Armed Forces Epidemiological Board. They submitted a report containing the following conclusions and recommendations [15]:

• There is strong support for the ultimate destruction of viable smallpox stocks in all repositories.
• However, in the face of evidence of a public health threat posed by the potential use of unregistered stocks of smallpox as an agent of terrorism or biological warfare, destruction should be deferred until specific information is obtained on the following three critical issues:

– The efficacy of currently available antiviral drugs.
– The efficacy of current and new cell-culture-derived vaccine preparations for the prevention of smallpox induced by high-dose aerosol challenge.
– Development and validation of potential animal models for the purpose of evaluating antivirals and new or improved vaccines.

• A short-term, focused research program to obtain this information should be established using the resources of CDC and the U.S. Army Medical Research Institute of Infectious Diseases (USAMRIID).
• If the proposed research program cannot be given sufficient priority for the work to be carried out within a reasonable period of time—3 to 5 years—this should be taken as an indication that neither the research nor the variola virus stocks are needed.

• Elimination of existing smallpox stocks would lessen but not eliminate the public health threat of orthopox disease. Consequently, the United States must establish and maintain a strong diagnosis and disease prevention effort.

DHHS and DOD also created a Joint Coordinating Group (JCG) to address critical scientific issues associated with destruction of variola virus stocks and to elaborate a research agenda involving collaboration among CDC, USAMRIID, the National Institutes of Health (NIH), and the U.S. Food and Drug Administration (FDA). The JCG identified three principal areas for research that encompassed the issues raised by the advisory group [21]. The first, dealing with antiviral substances, involves evaluation of treatment of smallpox with antiviral agents that have been approved by FDA for other purposes or are well on the way toward approval. The enormous costs of drug development, as well as the time involved, dictate the need to restrict the screening to these drugs. An initial step would be to undertake a screening of these compounds in cell cultures infected with variola virus or other orthopoxviruses and then to proceed through animal models using appropriate surrogate orthopoxviruses, recognizing that there is no satisfactory animal model for variola infection (see Chapter 6). A second research area identified by the JCG involves ascertaining the possible applicability of a model using monkeypox virus infection in monkeys to measure the effect of antivirals and assess the efficacy of vaccines. It was suggested that if this model were to prove unsatisfactory, further consideration would have to be given to the possible development of an animal model for smallpox, such as genetically modified rodents or immunosuppressed animals. Finally, the JCG noted the need to develop simple, rapid laboratory methods for identifying and differentiating among the various orthopoxviruses.

## RESEARCH AT CDC AND USAMRIID

In addition to sequencing of variola virus isolates at CDC, collaborative studies at CDC and USAMRIID have pursued the research program outlined by the JCG. Antiviral studies have included screening of drugs for inhibition of variola and other orthopoxviruses in cell culture and for protection against monkeypox in macaque monkeys, an animal model system considered to be more closely analogous to smallpox in humans than is vaccinia infection in monkeys. Several new drugs being developed for other medical problems have shown potential. Cidofovir, a DNA polymerase inhibitor, has been found to be active when used systemically in a murine model of vaccinia infection [22], to be topically and systemically effective against molluscum contagiosum [23], and to protect monkeys when treatment was initiated within 2 days following monkeypox virus exposure [24]. However, these results do not guarantee that the drug will provide protection against smallpox in humans. Imitosol, for example, inhibits cytomegalovirus (CMV) in humans, but not in guinea pigs or mice, the surrogate models of choice. Furthermore, cidofovir has significant side effects and must be injected intravenously with probenecid following hydration [24]. For these reasons, cidofovir appears unlikely to be an effective therapeutic agent for routine use against smallpox.

A DOD vaccine derived in cell culture using plaque-purified Connaught smallpox vaccine as seed virus was also tested under this program. Monkeys vaccinated with the DOD vaccine or commercially available vaccine were subsequently exposed to aerosolized monkeypox virus. Both the DOD vaccine and the commercial vaccine partially protected the monkeys against monkeypox infection [25]. Again, however, this finding cannot be considered conclusive. Although such experiments cannot be done for ethical reasons, there is no substitute for challenging the target host with live virus to prove protective efficacy [25].

For rapid diagnosis, CDC and USAMRIID have incorporated fluorescence-based polymerase chain reaction (PCR) technology in a suitcase-sized device that can identify and distinguish among the poxviruses. The assay is accurate with DNA prepared in the laboratory, but has not been proven with clinical materials in the field. Additional long-distance PCR techniques and restriction endonuclease assays that amplify and identify the entire genome have been developed. There are no routine serological assays that can specifically identify and differentiate variola virus antibodies in sera [26].

# PART III

♦ ♦ ♦ ♦ ♦

# Scientific Needs for Variola Virus

# 6

# Development of Antiviral Agents

The most compelling reason for continued retention of live variola stocks is the identification and development of antiviral agents for use in the event of a large outbreak of smallpox. As noted earlier, virtually the entire human population is now susceptible to smallpox. Depending on the size, density, and mobility of the exposed population and the means by which the virus was introduced, millions of individuals could quickly become or be at risk of becoming infected.

There is no known drug therapy available that is effective in the treatment of smallpox. There is also no diagnostic test capable of detecting infected individuals during the incubation period preceding clinical symptoms. Vaccination can reduce the seriousness of the disease if administered within 4 days of infection [1]. However, the current U.S. vaccine supply is limited and may be deteriorating. Moreover, if an outbreak were to occur in a highly mobile population, widespread immunization within this narrow time frame would be logistically challenging. Antiviral medications with prophylactic and/or therapeutic properties—especially those that were safe, could be mass produced, exhibited good shelf life at ambient temperature, and could be taken orally—would therefore be critical in dealing with a large-scale outbreak of smallpox. Access to live variola virus would make it possible to test the activity of candidate antivirals in cell culture and could ultimately lead to the development of novel animal models systems for testing antivariola activity in vivo. It must be recognized however that neither of these preclinical approaches is able to substitute completely for trials conducted in infected patients. The combination of extensive preclinical studies with clinical pharmacokinetic data nevertheless provides a credible strategy for estimating the best dosing regimen to combat an outbreak of smallpox in unvaccinated humans.

## IN VITRO ASSAYS

The discovery of antiviral agents is currently an active field of research in academia and in the biotechnology and pharmaceutical industries [27]. More than 20 new chemical and biological agents have received U.S. Food and Drug Administration approval for treatment of human viral diseases in the last 10 years. Numerous compounds, recombinant proteins, and monoclonal antibodies are currently under active investigation as antiviral or immune-boosting agents. Some but not all antiviral agents have been tested for their ability to prevent variola virus infection of cultured cells in the Biological Safety Level 4 (BSL-4) biological containment facilities at the Centers for Disease Control and Prevention (CDC) in Atlanta or the State Center of Virology and Biotechnology (VECTOR) in Kotsovo.*

Cidofovir, for example, is an antiviral, initially developed as a DNA polymerase inhibitor for the treatment of cytomegalovirus (CMV) retinitis, then found to be active in preventing variola infection of cultured cells (see also Chapter 5). While cidofovir's low oral bioavailability and potential for severe renal toxicity limit its clinical utility for the treatment of variola infection, numerous advances in drug discovery technology—such as combinatorial chemistry, molecular modeling, and high-throughput screening—are providing many new chemical entities that could be tested for their safety and efficacy against variola [27, 28]. Moreover, successful strategies for blocking the infectivity of other types of viruses may suggest new approaches for combating variola. If a large outbreak of smallpox is a credible threat, the infrastructure for testing the antivariola activity of existing and future antiviral agents must be retained by CDC on an ongoing basis. Should a backlog of promising agents develop, expansion of the infrastructure might well be considered.

Discovery of a new antiviral agent is a complex and costly process, typically requiring evaluation of many tens of thousands of candidates in several assays. The primary screening assay typically tests the ability of an agent to bind and inactivate a recombinant, cell-free target protein of viral or human origin, or inhibit replication of the virus itself. Intrinsic potency is determined at this stage in titration experiments, while measurement of potency against closely related proteins provides an indication of specificity. Since single amino acid changes can have dramatic effects on the potency and specificity of antiviral agents, it is imperative that authentic target proteins be tested. Authentication of the target protein includes sequence analysis of the corresponding DNA from several clinical isolates.

The potency and efficacy of an antiviral agent are influenced by many factors in addition to the agent's ability to bind to the target protein. These factors include

---

*John W. Huggins, Personal communication, December 1998.

(but are by no means limited to) the intracellular and/or extracellular location of the target protein, the ability of agents to permeate host cells in the case of intracellular targets, the local concentration and turnover rate of the target protein within the infected cell, and conformational changes that may be induced within the target protein by neighboring proteins if the target is part of a protein complex. These latter considerations require that candidate antivirals be tested in cell culture assays employing live virus so that potency and efficacy in this more complex setting can be estimated. The concentration of agent required to block infectivity by 90 percent in cell culture ($IC_{90}$) is often a valuable guide to determining the concentration of agent that must be continuously maintained in vivo in order to obtain the desired therapeutic effect. To the extent that animal model studies are problematic (see the following section), cell culture assays provide the only preclinical opportunity to evaluate the ability of an agent to block host cell infection. Moreover, even if animal model systems are available, cell culture assays provide the only preclinical opportunity to test the activity on human cells.

Whenever possible, orthopoxvirus family members other than variola should be used for routine testing involving live virus in order to reduce the hazards associated with handling of variola by laboratory staff. This is particularly true if the target protein is identical among orthopoxvirus family members. Another strategy would be to inactivate a gene that variola requires for replication. This gene would necessarily be unrelated to the gene whose protein product is the drug target. Because replication-defective virus is able to replicate only in host cells genetically engineered to express the viral gene, the risk to laboratory personnel and the likelihood of an outbreak originating from a laboratory would be significantly reduced.

Although useful for general drug screening, however, use of such recombinants has limitations. In particular, such genetically engineered host cell lines are not necessarily representative of cells infected by the virus in vivo. It is therefore essential that candidate agents be tested for activity and potency in a tissue culture assay employing clinical isolates of variola virus and recently isolated human cells to ascertain whether equivalent potency is obtained in the surrogate system.

Evidence supporting this contention comes from studies showing that a given antiviral agent can exhibit substanitally different potencies against related viruses in tissue culture. For example, non-nucleoside reverse transcriptase inhibitors (e.g., nevaripine, delavirdine, and efavirenz) are active agents against human immunodeficiency virus 1 (HIV-1), but not HIV-2; likewise, amantadine and rimantadine are active against influenza A, but not influenza B, while sorivudine is very effective against herpes simplex virus 1 (HSV-1), but ineffective against HSV-2 [29–31]. Even more relevant is the observation that phosphonates related to cidofovir are about fivefold more active against variola in culture than against either monkeypox or cowpox in culture.* Assay of these substances against either cowpox or monkeypox would therefore result in a substantial underestimation of their potency against variola. Underestimation of potency could lead to overdosage; greater risk of toxicity; and the need for larger, more costly inventories of antiviral drugs. On the other hand, overestimation of potency could encourage selection of escape mutants. In addition, it is highly desirable and accepted practice that in vitro testing be conducted with several clinical isolates of variola to ensure that results obtained with a given isolate are representative of the species, if not the genus of *Orthopoxviridae*.

## ANIMAL MODELS

The activity of antiviral agents is influenced by their pharmacokinetic and metabolic profiles, which are examined initially through studies conducted on uninfected animals. Regimens of increasing single and multiple doses are used to determine drug absorption and duration, tolerance, and maximum tolerated dose. The $IC_{90}$ determined in vitro using live variola virus and cultured human host cells as described above would be used, along with observed blood and tissue levels of antiviral agent in test animals, to design a dose-ranging study aimed at determining safety and tolerability in humans under an approved investigational new drug (IND) application. This is essentially the approach taken to develop antiviral agents for the treatment of HIV.

While experience with the development of anti-HIV drugs is instructive with respect to the development of antivariola agents, there are no patients infected with variola with whom to conduct pharmacodynamic and efficacy studies. Animal model studies therefore provide the only opportunity to study the pharmacodynamic effects of a candidate antiviral agent in a whole-animal setting. Specifically, it is important to determine prior to use during a large-scale human outbreak what effect the agent has on the natural history of the disease, the development of immunity, and the clearance of virus when given before and during various stages of infection. Once again, the lack of an animal model specific to variola virus means that use of other orthopoxvirus family members should be considered, especially if the agent has demonstrated similar activity against other family members in cell culture. Priority would reasonably be given to antivariola agents whose activity against other orthopoxviruses would permit their evaluation in surrogate animal model systems. To the extent that otherwise promising agents exhibited variable potency against different orthopoxviruses in

---

*These include for cidofovir: 3–5 micromolar for variola compared with 15 micromolar for cowpox and monkeypox; for HPMPA 5 micromolar compared with 30 micromolar; and for PMEA 3 micromolar compared with 30 micromolar. John W. Huggins, Personal communication, December 1998.

cell culture, it would be highly desirable to develop models using variola itself such that the pharmacodynamic properties of variola-specific compounds could also be assessed. Regulatory agencies such as the U.S. Food and Drug Administration should be active in the development of such drugs for use in emergencies.

> **BOX 6-1 Animal Models**
>
> There have been several attempts to develop suitable animal models to study variola virus infection. Primates used have included Cynomolgus monkeys (*Macaca irus*), rhesus monkeys (*Macaca mulatta*), bonnet monkeys (*Macaca radiata*), orangutans and chimpanzees. However, variola virus infections in these animals do have the same features and effects typical of human infections, such as dissemination throughout the body, fever, rash, and/or death. Hence, there is no known animal model suitable for studying the pathogenesis of variola virus in humans.
>
> Although not perfectly comparable, the effectiveness of antiviral agents in combating monkeypox virus infections in monkeys has been used in lieu of direct variola virus challenge because that disease in monkeys is similar to smallpox in humans. However, it must be recognized that even in this surrogate model, there is considerable uncertainty regarding the degree of extrapolation of such factors as regimen, effective dose, and timing to variola in humans. This uncertainty stems from intrinsic differences between monkey and human hosts, as well as between the monkeypox and variola viruses.
>
> Two aspects of variola infection are key to understanding the pathogenesis of the virus: (1) the interactions with the immune system and (2) the mechanisms governing dissemination of the virus throughout the body. In principle, it is possible to develop a suitable animal model system for studying the mechanism of variola dissemination, as well as to introduce critical elements of the human immune system into experimental animals, such as mice, in order to study variola virus interactions with the immune system. Although rapid progress has been made in recent years with these techniques, these approaches are not yet possible.
>
> More work would therefore have to be done on these reconstituted systems before they could be used for routine testing of antivirals and vaccines.

# 7

# Development of Vaccines

Vaccination within 3 to 4 days of exposure to smallpox is an important control strategy that prevents the disease or modifies its severity. In addition to adequate supplies of vaccine, a large-scale outbreak would necessitate well-defined plans for their rapid distribution and inoculation of those exposed to or at risk of exposure to variola virus.

The administration of live vaccinia vaccine made possible the global eradication of smallpox in the 1970s. The clinical experience with vaccinia vaccine is vast, involving millions of recipients who were immunized over a period of many decades in all geographic areas of the world, often at times and locations in which health conditions were far from optimal [1]. Given this broad experience, variola virus is not needed in the maintenance of vaccine prevention capabilities. However, the most important concern related to vaccine prevention of smallpox is that the available supplies of vaccinia vaccine are limited and may be deteriorating because of prolonged storage. This situation must be addressed if the reemergence of smallpox is considered to be a risk or if laboratory research using live variola virus is to be continued.

The vaccinia vaccines made from virus isolates that were used so widely against smallpox in the past are accepted as being relatively safe and highly effective, as long as proper standards for their manufacture, storage, and delivery are maintained. The testing of new lots of vaccinia vaccine made using standard methods, or of well-characterized strains of vaccinia grown in tissue culture cells, would not require live variola virus. Although not of overriding concern, retention of live variola virus stocks would, however, permit corroborating assessments of the probable efficacy of new tissue culture vaccines, using laboratory assays to measure immune inhibition of variola replication or testing against variola challenge in animal models not yet available. Moreover, the development of novel smallpox vaccines not incorporating live vaccinia might be undertaken in order to provide vaccines safe for use with immunocompromised individuals (see the discussion below). Variola virus would have to be available for the later phases of evaluation of any such novel vaccines before their clinical use could be considered.

## CURRENT STATUS OF VACCINIA VACCINE PREPARATIONS

The commercial smallpox vaccine currently approved for use in the United States is a lyophilized preparation of live vaccinia virus prepared from calf lymph. The vaccine is made by inoculating animals with seed virus derived from the New York City Board of Health (NYCBH) strain of vaccinia [32]. Vaccinia vaccine made using this traditional process in animals can be evaluated for potency by demonstrating reactogenicity or "take," defined by formation of the characteristic lesion at the site of inoculation by skin abrasion.

These vaccines exhibit high seroconversion rates and infrequent adverse events. For every 1 million individuals inoculated, 75 experienced medical complications from the vaccine [1]. Possible complications include generalized vaccinia, which in persons without underlying illness is characterized by a vesicular rash of varying extent that generally is self-limiting and requires little or no therapy. Postvaccinal encephalitis is the most serious complication in otherwise healthy individuals. It generally affects infants less than 1 year old, and is associated with a mortality rate of about 25 percent and a risk of permanent neurologic consequences in about 25 percent of its survivors. Persons with eczema or exfoliative skin conditions may experience a disseminated or systemic infection (eczema vaccinatum). Finally, progressive vaccinia is a severe, potentially fatal illness that occurs almost exclusively among persons with cellular immunodeficiency. The HIV epidemic and the new immune-modulating drugs and therapies currently used to treat cancers and allow successful transplantation of organs and bone marrow have placed many people worldwide at risk of this complication. The limited experience with vaccinia vaccines in those with HIV infection (two military personnel inoculated before being identified as HIV-positive) suggests that use of the vaccine with those individuals is likely to produce disseminated vaccinia infection [33, 34]. The largest problem is likely to be in countries with substantial prevalence of HIV infection.

Vaccinia immune globulin (VIG) is the only product developed for the treatment of complications of vaccinia vaccination. VIG is effective for the treatment of eczema vaccinatum and some cases of progressive vaccinia; it is of no benefit in the treatment of postvaccinal encephalitis.

Wyeth Laboratories, currently the only licensed producer of vaccinia vaccine in the United States, discontinued distribution of smallpox vaccine to civilians in 1983 [35]. Since then, CDC has been the only nonmilitary source of the Wyeth vaccine and the only distributor of VIG. CDC maintains the vaccinia under contract with Wyeth, while Baxter-Highland Laboratories maintains VIG for the U.S. Department of Defense. In the past, CDC has maintained a supply of several million doses of vaccinia vaccine and the requisite VIG for treating complications. However, these supplies are now 17 to 20 years old and exhibit signs of loss of potency.

Recently, some of the stored vaccinia diluent vaccine was found to be unusable. Without assessing the entire supply, it is not possible to know exactly how many usable doses are currently available. Replacing these vaccine doses is problematic because the cost of undertaking the manufacture of new lots of vaccine and completing the applications required to obtain government approval of these preparations is high enough to discourage commercial enterprises from doing so. Moreover, manufacture of new vaccine to augment current stocks would have to meet current standards of vaccine production and standardization, which might require adjustments in the production process. In addition, no VIG is currently available. The license on the available VIG expired in October 1998, and the U.S. Food and Drug Administration (FDA) did not grant an extension. The status of the VIG stock is pending final review by FDA and Baxter-Highland Laboratories in early 1999.*

As noted above, the evaluation of new lots of live vaccinia vaccine would not require laboratory testing involving the use of live variola virus. During the history of smallpox vaccination, many different vaccinia isolates and several different animal hosts were used to manufacture vaccine. These diverse vaccines were effective against epidemiologically distinct variola viruses responsible for smallpox outbreaks that were separated by distance as well as time. In practice, however, testing of the reactogenicity of new lots of vaccinia, even if performed under standard conditions, requires access to VIG. The availability of VIG, which is made by immunizing healthy human donors with vaccinia vaccine, would enable a therapeutic intervention in the unlikely event of an adverse response. Thus the lack of VIG is a further obstacle to replenishing the vaccinia vaccine supply.

## EVALUATION OF VACCINIA VACCINE DERIVED FROM TISSUE CULTURE

In replacing the existing supplies of vaccinia vaccine or planning for a potential situation in which widespread vaccination might be required, one could make the vaccine by infecting tissue culture cells, rather than by inoculating animals. The current approach to the manufacture of most other live attenuated vaccines is based on growth of the vaccine virus in tissue culture cells that have

---

* John Becker, Personal communication, December 1998.

been certified for production of human vaccines. Some limited evaluation of the safety and immunogenicity, or potency to produce immunity, of vaccinia vaccine made in tissue culture has been carried out in susceptible individuals in Japan [1]. Similar vaccines have been produced in Germany and The Netherlands, but vaccine preparations of this type have not been approved for use in the United States.

Vaccinia vaccines made in tissue culture cells are closely related to those made in animals because the same virus stocks, such as the NYCBH strain, can be used. As noted earlier, given the predicted similarities between new and traditional vaccinia vaccines, the validation of new vaccines derived from tissue culture would not require the use of variola virus. Comparisons of genomic stability could be made to confirm the relationship of vaccinia derived after replication in these cells to the input virus and to vaccinia preparations made by inoculating animals. Molecular analyses of vaccines produced in this manner could be used to document the preservation of the expected vaccinia genotype by comparison with existing vaccinia vaccine stocks. The potency of vaccinia vaccines made in tissue culture cells could be assessed in human volunteers using the protocols for testing of reactogenicity and seroconversion that are used for standard vaccinia vaccines. Vaccines made in this way would be closely related to existing vaccines and could be evaluated using "bridging" studies. In such studies, the new vaccine is compared with the existing vaccine in small numbers of healthy susceptible individuals, using assays for vaccine reactogenicity or "take" and seroconversion that have served as markers of effective vaccinia vaccines in the past.

These measures of equivalence between vaccines derived from tissue culture and traditional vaccines made in animals would not, however, constitute definitive proof of protective efficacy, which would have to be defined by field testing under conditions of natural exposure. No specific immunologic correlates of protection for vaccinia vaccines were defined during the smallpox era. Licensure of vaccinia vaccines derived from tissue culture would therefore require a departure from the usual criteria for regulatory approval. Nevertheless, there would be a high degree of confidence in predictions of efficacy based on direct comparison of the vaccines thus derived and existing vaccine with regard to local reactogenicity and immunogenicity. This judgment is based on the fact that limited passage of vaccinia in tissue culture cells would not be likely to cause further attenuation, and preservation of the capacity of the vaccine strain to replicate in vivo could be documented by the expected lesion formation after abrasive inoculation. It should be noted that use of an alternative route of inoculation, such as subcutaneous injection, would eliminate the latter important correlate of potency and hamper the judgment of vaccine equivalence. As suggested above, although it is not an overriding concern, retention of live variola virus would permit complementary or corroborating assessments of the probable efficacy of new vaccines derived from tissue culture, using laboratory assays to measure immune inhibition of variola replication or testing against variola challenge in animal models (assuming suitable animal models became available).

## EVALUATION OF NOVEL VACCINES

As noted earlier, clinical experience with vaccinia vaccines demonstrates that assessment of the level of viral attenuation measured in animals is not sufficient to prevent the occurrence of disseminated vaccinia in some individuals with compromised immune responses [32]. Thus novel vaccines might be developed to provide safe vaccination of these populations. Manufacturing the vaccine in tissue culture would not be expected to alter the risks of vaccinating immunocompromised individuals. To ensure safety, it would be necessary to develop vaccines that contained no live vaccinia virus or were made from vaccinia strains that had been changed genetically to block their ability to spread after inoculation. Options include subunit protein vaccines, DNA vaccines, synthesis of noninfectious particles, and others. Laboratory and animal testing in yet-to-be-devised systems would also be necessary.

Scientifically, the task of developing novel vaccines that would be safe and effective against smallpox in immunocompromised patients would not be straightforward. A priori, it can be predicted to be an extremely costly effort, requiring years to accomplish. In fact, development of such vaccines may not be feasible because the varied immune deficiencies of different patients at risk may prevent an adequate response to any generic candidate vaccine. During the smallpox era, several highly attenuated strains of vaccinia virus were obtained by passage in tissue culture, and it is known that repeatedly growing vaccinia in minced chick embryo cells reduces the virulence of the virus in subsequent generations [1]. However, the genetic basis for this attenuation of virulence is not known, and whether these strains are safe or effective as vaccines for individuals who have abnormal immune systems is uncertain.

The efficacy of any vaccine that was substantially changed in design could not be established by direct comparison with traditional vaccinia vaccines without more complete understanding of protection against variola immunopathogenesis. Confidence in the efficacy of different preparations of live vaccinia vaccines is based on the fact that these vaccines contain the complete virus, and the virus causes a limited infection in the vaccinated person. As a result, the immune system becomes sensitized to many viral proteins, and many memory B cells and T cells that can recognize cognate smallpox virus antigens are generated. Novel vaccines that departed from this design could not be judged for potency based on the criterion of reactogenicity at the inoculation site or by genetic comparison with vaccinia, and there are no known specific immunologic correlates of protection against smallpox.

Much of the initial work toward developing new smallpox vaccines could be done without the use of variola virus. For example, persons given candidate novel vaccines could be evaluated using assays demonstrating the induction of immunity. Variola proteins expressed from plasmids or in other vectors could be used to detect variola-specific immunity, such as neutralizing antibodies or other viral proteins, or recognition of variola proteins by T cells that mediate cytotoxicity and antigen-specific cytokine release. Nevertheless, confirmatory assessment of the induction of functional protective immunity would require testing using variola virus, and the margin of confidence in the probable efficacy of such vaccines would be enhanced by studies of challenge by variola virus in animal models yet to be developed.

Despite the major obstacles involved, the design of novel vaccines is scientifically feasible, and may constitute a rationale for preserving variola stocks for future use in such an endeavor. From a public health perspective, however, circumstances that would require vaccination of immunocompromised persons might never arise. If an early, limited outbreak were to be detected, it should be possible to protect these individuals and keep them from becoming new source cases by vaccinating a large enough portion of the population to prevent spread of the infection to those who could not be immunized safely. Should a very large-scale, contemporaneous exposure occur, protective isolation would be the only alternative to vaccination. If large numbers of people were placed at risk, protective isolation would not be a practical strategy, and a noninfectious vaccine would be valuable. On the other hand, one can envision an exposure situation evolving so rapidly that immunocompromised patients within the population at large could not be identified and excluded from the vaccine campaign in a timely manner. It is important to recognize that under these conditions, the availability of a novel vaccine safe for high-risk patients would have limited practical benefit.

# 8

# Detection and Diagnosis

The term "detection" is used here to denote identification of the virus in the environment, while "diagnosis" refers to determination that the virus or pathogen has infected a human host. The need to detect variola virus could arise as a result of experimentation with the virus under BSL-4 conditions in well-controlled laboratories, but is perhaps more likely to occur as a result of experimentation with unregistered variola virus under less optimal conditions. Detection technology could provide additional safety by offering proof of containment if research were to be conducted on live variola virus. Exposure to variola virus could also result from the intended or unintended action of a terrorist individual or group or the planned action of a rogue state. Should such an event occur, timely environmental detection and early diagnosis of human infection would be extremely valuable.

The development of sensitive and specific detection and diagnostic strategies would probably involve identification of variola virus nucleic acid or protein. Such approaches would be dependent on knowledge of the range of variability in natural variola sequences and/or the sequences of their encoded proteins. It is likely that from current knowledge of the sequences of individual orthopoxvirus genes and from the complete sequences of three variola major virus isolates that are available, polymerase chain reaction (PCR) primer pairs capable of differentially amplifying DNA segments from all previously sequenced orthopoxviruses could be selected.

Such primers would probably be valid for the sensitive detection of any variola virus. The sequencing of additional strains of variola virus DNA from dispersed geographic origins, however, would provide an additional margin of validity with minimal additional risk or cost. Sequences that are unique to variola virus have greater potential for variability among different strains than sequences that are common to the orthopoxvirus family. Therefore, additional sequencing of variola virus samples is critically important for development of the nucleic acid detection technology needed to identify variola virus, as opposed to other orthopoxviruses. There is no guarantee that an emerging strain would be represented in the archive, but understanding of the variation would assist in determining the relation of the new strain to known isolates. Moreover, the specific identification of variola virus would be a necessary feature of detection or diagnosis of variola virus infection should the precise source of the infection be unknown. The two variola major isolates that have been sequenced come from India and Bangladesh, within or near the Indian subcontinent, and one variola minor isolate comes from Brazil. The degree of similarity between these variola virus sequences and those of strains of variola from other parts of the world is unknown. Research on this issue—including sequencing of the entire genome or selected genome segments of additional isolates, or extended PCR and restriction fragment length polymorphism (RFLP) assay of entire genome DNA—should move forward as rapidly as possible.

It may be noted that additional sequencing and PCR/RFLP assay of other orthopoxvirus DNA sequences may be important for specificity issues. This is especially true for monkeypox virus DNA. Little is known about the range of DNA sequence variability among isolates of monkeypox virus.

Concerns analogous to those regarding DNA sequence conservation and variability would hold for protein- or antibody-based detection or diagnostic strategies. Some work on validating target sequences for sensitive or specific detection or diagnosis has been done at CDC and at VECTOR. The current state of that work needs to be critically assessed.

## ENVIRONMENTAL DETECTION

Environmental detection would involve instrumentation for sampling the environment. For example, a vacuum system with a contained filter trap could be developed for air sampling, and various adsorbents could be prepared for surface sampling. For the most part, any orthopoxvirus could be used in place of variola virus to devise suitable sampling techniques, assuming similar biophysical characteristics and stability (as appears to be the case). However, variola virus or possibly another live orthopoxvirus expressing variola virus surface protein(s) or containing variola virus DNA might be essential for final testing of a detection technology and strategy. For example, a filter coated with a variola-specific monoclonal antibody might trap variola virus. Identification of the virus might then rely on PCR for DNA testing or a second antibody for antigen testing. A solely protein-based detection assay, such as those using monoclonal antibodies in antigen capture, would be relatively insensitive, but might be faster

## DETECTION AND DIAGNOSIS

and more portable. Another live orthopoxvirus containing one or a few variola virus genes would be preferable to live variola virus for final test validation because of safety concerns. However, current policies prohibit the making of recombinant poxviruses containing any variola virus gene(s), and it is conceivable that variola proteins expressed in such a recombinant might not exhibit authentic structural and functional properties.

Furthermore, little is known about the surface proteins of variola. Detection is based solely on surface components of other orthopoxviruses that are extrapolated to variola components. This extrapolation is based on predictions that depend on the homology of the corresponding DNA of these surface proteins and those of variola virus. Limited biochemical studies of variola surface proteins would therefore be valuable. These studies could be conducted prior to destruction of the virus stocks.

One alternative might be to construct a variola virus recombinant that was incapable of replicating in normal human cells and to use such a recombinant for test validation under highly restricted conditions. Altering the regulations to permit limited insertion of part or all of a variola virus gene into vaccinia virus would be preferable to undertaking work with a host-range-restricted variola virus recombinant. Nonetheless, there would still be considerable security and safety concerns associated with using an almost complete variola virus. Moreover, the rigorous testing needed to prove the authenticity of the protein structure and function of a host-range mutant might make such an approach time-consuming and excessively expensive.

## DIAGNOSIS OF INFECTION

Sensitive diagnosis of variola virus infection at the earliest stages would most likely be accomplished using some form of nucleic acid amplification technology to detect variola in saliva, sputum, blood, or lymphatic aspiration. However, initial epidemiological or medical interventions might be indicated solely upon finding orthopoxvirus-specific nucleic acid in human material in a setting in which variola virus infection was a possibility. Although technology for detecting antibodies to variola virus would be of limited or no utility in the first few days after exposure, robust antibody detection schemes might be highly useful for epidemiological surveillance following an outbreak.

Use of host-specific components—for example, in blood, saliva, or urine—to screen for variola virus upon early indications of infection might be feasible were the pathogenesis of variola better understood. IgM (immunoglobulin M) antibodies might be detectable within 2 weeks of exposure and IgG antibodies within 3 to 4 weeks of exposure. Detection of antibodies may be less expensive, more portable, and more stable than detection of nucleic acid or antigen. Rapid and safe type-specific bedside tests would be useful in the event of potential variola infection.

Diagnostic strategies could be verified using mouse or subhuman primate models of orthopoxvirus infection. A recombinant vaccinia virus carrying all or part of a variola virus gene would be useful for a step in the validation, subject to the concerns expressed above with regard to detection strategies. Research with a vaccinia virus construct carrying a single variola gene would not be constrained by the need to work in BSL-4 facilities. Some parallel work with monkeypox virus diagnostics in monkey models would be desirable to validate ease of detection in the context of an analogous primate virus-host model.

## ALTERNATIVES TO LIVE VIRUS

The development of detection and diagnostic strategies would not require live variola virus per se, beyond the need for additional recombinant DNA stocks and sequencing. Much of the developmental in vitro research could be done with isolated recombinant variola virus DNA and recombinant produced protein. The requirement for virus for field epidemiological detection, for particle stability verification, and for diagnostic test validation in experimental models could be bypassed by using vaccinia virus as a representative of the orthopoxvirus family. A vaccinia virus recombinant containing all or part of the relevant variola virus DNA segment would be useful for the validation of tests in appropriate epidemiological or experimental animal infection model systems, although assessment of the authenticity of the recombinant as compared with live variola virus would be needed. Parallel work with monkeypox virus might add a small margin of additional validation.

# 9

# Bioinformatics

Although possession of the viral genome sequence does not yield total knowledge about the integrated biology, virulence, or transmissibility of a virus, much can be learned from a variety of studies based on these sequences. An important question is the variability of genetic information (DNA sequence) among different isolates of the virus obtained from patients in different geographic locations, although available collections are not well-ordered sets of variola virus strains. Multiple clones or PCR products should be sequenced to assess diversity. Significant differences are known to exist between the sequences of variola major and minor, but the extent of the variation and the importance of the identified differences for virulence in each of the two subspecies or even within individual isolates have not been determined [36]. The extent and consistency of sequence variability might provide essential clues to the pathogenesis, virulence, and evolution of the virus and the nature of the infection. For example, a recent outbreak of monkeypox exhibited somewhat greater human-to-human transmission than had been the case in the past. However, preliminary results from sequencing of DNA fragments of monkeypox virus isolates obtained at various times since 1970 suggest that the virus has changed very little over this period. Thus at present, there is no clear evidence that the rate of human-to-human transmission of monkeypox is likely to increase [37]. DNA sequence information from a characteristic set of variola virus isolates could enhance our capability to assess whether human monkeypox is evolving transmission characteristics similar to those of smallpox. Variola virus stocks need to be retained until a sufficient number have been cloned, or PCR amplifications have been obtained and analyzed.

## VARIABILITY OF VARIOLA VIRUS

While the complete genomic sequences of a few variola virus isolates are available, the overall scope of such information remains limited. As noted in Chapter 5, the complete genome DNA of variola major virus Bangladesh-1975 (GenBank #L22579) has been sequenced from clones with about sixfold redundancy. The variola major virus India-1967 (GenBank X69198) genome, except for a small region at each DNA terminal, and the variola minor alastrim virus Brazil-1966 genome (EMBL Y167080) also have been sequenced, with about twofold redundancy. The samples in the CDC and VECTOR repositories do not, however, represent a complete archive of characterized strains from the different outbreaks in recent history.*

Although the sequences of the above strains are not entirely identical, they are nearly so. Direct sequence comparison of the Bangladesh-1975 and India-1967 strains shows that the viruses are 99.2 percent identical throughout the entire genome (see Figure 9-1) [6, 36, 38]. While in one sense this finding argues for relatively little variability, that conclusion should be tempered by the following considerations. Most of the differences are clustered in the terminal regions of the viral genome. Those regions contain genes that frequently are not essential for viral replication, yet typically are associated with pathogenesis, interact with the immune system, and affect virulence and host range. While only 18 of 200 proteins in the entire genome differ significantly between the Bangladesh and India strains, 7 of 30 open reading frames at the left terminus and 8 of 22 open reading frames near the right terminus show variation between the two viruses [36]. It must be remembered that a very minor change—a single base addition or deletion or a single amino acid coded by a gene—can lead to profound effects in the corresponding proteins that determine variations in virulence. Moreover, available sequence data have been derived from plaque-purified isolates whose DNA was cloned into plasmids, and there are sparse or no data on heterogeneity within individual isolates, the effect of cloning in bacteria, or the heterogeneity in strains other than those discussed above.

The issue of heterogeneity can be addressed using different strategies, such as multiple plaque-purified clones from the same isolate, or a complete catalogue of sequences from the left and right terminal regions of the genomes from strains with quite different clinical histories or epidemiological descriptions. Limited studies have shown that long-distance PCR and RFLP analysis of specific amplifications occasionally does not produce the restriction pattern predicted in the published sequence obtained from cloned DNA fragments [26, 39–41]. Specifically, within one PCR-amplified fragment where, say, four restriction sites with a given enzyme would have been predicted, only three are found with the corresponding adjustments in size. This discrepancy may be the result of poor long-distance PCR copy fidelity, unappreciated heterogeneity within the

---

* Joseph J. Esposito, Personal communication, December 1998.

DNA, or sequencing errors introduced because clones were used to determine the sequence. The uncertainty inherent in this analytic method and cloning in plasmids reinforces the importance of examining a large set of isolates to develop consensus on the DNA molecular preparation. Sequencing provides only a snapshot of the virus genome, which actually exists in nature as a molecular array.

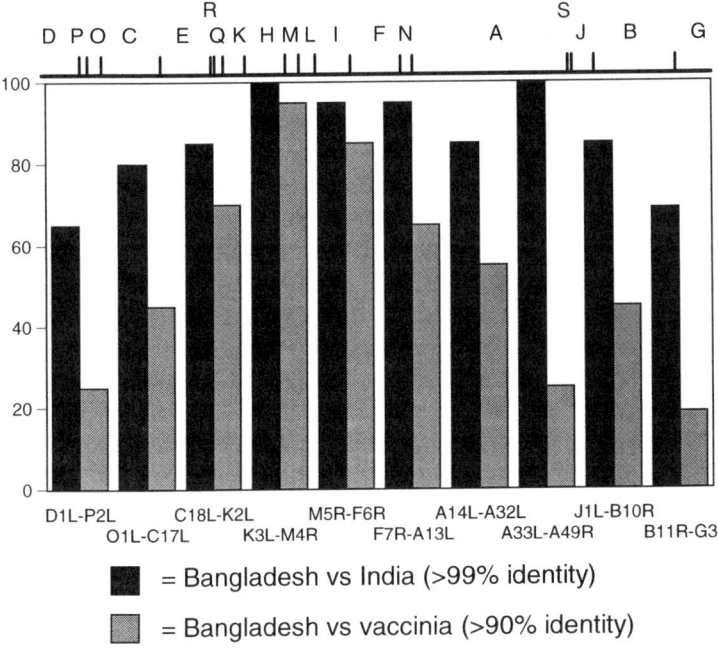

**FIGURE 9-1** This figure illustrates the degree of conservation and variation between the Bangladesh (BSH) and India (IND) strains and between vaccinia and BSH by considering, on the Hind III genome map, the percent amino acid identity of predicted proteins. The open reading frames (ORF) were divided into 10 groups of 20 ORF across the genome, and the percentage of BSH and IND ORF that encode proteins of >99 percent amino acid sequence identity was determined. The analysis showed that the most varied proteins arise from the DNA terminal regions. Interestingly, the group of ORF A14L–A32L encodes proteins with greater amino acid diversity than does the group A33L–A49R, which is more proximal to the right end of the BSH and IND Hind III map. Also shown is a histogram that illustrates the striking difference in the amino acid sequence of proteins of vaccinia and BSH. SOURCE: Shchelkunov et al., Comparison of the genome DNA sequences of Bangladesh-1975 and India-1967 variola viruses. *Virus Research* 36:107–118, 1995. Copyright 1995, Elsevier Science; reprinted with permission.

## POTENTIAL DEVELOPMENTS

Information about the variations discussed above could be critical for the development of diagnostic reagents, subunit vaccines, and therapeutic drugs. It might also shed light on the mechanisms of viral virulence and host tropism. Much could be deduced about the degree of diversity and variation by sequencing the DNA from a comprehensive set of viral isolates. Long-distance, high-fidelity PCR would ideally be employed, with staggered initiation sites to produce overlapping sequences of sufficient redundancy to ensure the ability to determine the entire sequences with adequate accuracy. Such cloning and evaluation of sequence variability would necessarily have to be done before viral stocks were destroyed. Once sufficient DNA plasmid clones had been obtained and sequenced or analyzed by genome PCR or RFLP, live virus would no longer be required for most of the currently available informatics methods.

The open reading frames (ORF) of the smallpox virus genome have been identified in the genomes already sequenced. New sequences would help to identify naturally occurring variations and verify the validity of sequences already determined. Particular putative protein products could be studied from the perspective of the degree to which there was amino acid sequence conservation (or variation). Putative genes could be compared with equivalent ORF in other orthopoxviruses, as well as with ORF encoding similar proteins from the cell and in the genomes of other types of viruses. In particular, the ORF of the smallpox virus genome that are thought to be associated with virulence could be compared with those of other orthopoxviruses, including monkeypox virus, possibly leading to the identification of genes important for determining the pathogenicity, virulence, transmissibility, and human tropism of variola virus.

It has been reported that transfection of the intact vaccinia virus genome as DNA into cells infected with fowlpox virus leads to production of vaccinia virus [42]. Thus far, however, neither virion DNA fragments (representing the entire viral sequence) nor viral DNA from a plasmid has been successful in regenerating infectious vaccinia. This failure could be due to technical problems that might be solved as the technology improves. If so, it also should be possible to recreate live smallpox viruses from the DNA clones of overlapping fragments. This capability would have profound implications for issues of security, safety, and ethics surrounding the proposed destruction of live variola virus stocks. The ability to reconstitute viruses from DNA clones would make it possible to engineer a variety of attenuated viruses that would constitute an effective form of biological containment to help ensure safety while working with live virus.

Infectious poxviruses have not yet been created from assembled plasmids or synthetic DNA fragments, but there is no technical impediment to the eventual establishment of this ability. It is entirely possible that future advances in gene synthesis and transfection technologies would enable synthesis of variola virus from the published sequence information. There is no way of predicting the rate at which such technologies might develop.

# 10

# Understanding of the Biology of Variola Virus

As noted earlier, smallpox was eradicated prior to the modern age of cell and molecular biology, virology, and immunology. Therefore, the basics of viral replication, determinants of viral virulence, and pathogenesis of the disease are not as well understood as they are for other pathogens.

Since variola virus is a pathogen that is uniquely adapted to cause severe, widespread human illness, it is highly likely that it has evolved to specifically thwart an effective immune response to infection. Poxviruses are the largest of the viruses and produce many proteins that are not necessary for virus replication, but presumably enhance the ability of the virus to cause disease. The multiple mechanisms used by poxviruses to evade host immune responses, the unique proteins these viruses produce, and their interactions with the host are just beginning to be identified. As the database expands, questions about the interactions of variola virus with human cells and immune responses and about the functions of these disease-producing variola proteins will become more obvious and pressing. The ability to identify the interactions between variola virus and host proteins would likely provide new insights into important aspects of the human immune system that would not be apparent from studies of other viruses.

## VIRUS-CELL INTERACTIONS

Viruses adapt to their hosts in large part by evolving to interact efficiently with host cells in initiating infection and producing large amounts of virus. The virus spreads to different organs of the host and in this process causes tissue damage. Strains of a virus (e.g., variola major and variola minor) differ in their virulence or ability to cause fatal disease. The differences in virulence may be due to changes in the rapidity of virus replication and spread, the amounts of virus produced, the ability to damage the cells in which the virus replicates, or the ability to evade the immune response of the host. In addition, orthopoxvirus tissue tropism genes have been identified in vaccinia virus and cowpox (C7L, K1L, and CHOhr), and the morphogenesis of the multiple forms of orthopox-virus particles is becoming better understood [43, 44]. The genetic basis of orthopoxvirus infections may thereby be revealed. Infection of human cells grown in tissue culture could begin to provide answers to some of the following questions:

- Is there a unique molecule or series of molecules on the surface of human cells that makes them distinctly susceptible to infection with variola virus? What is the normal function of this molecule?
- How and in what order are the many genes of the virus expressed to produce viral proteins? Do these proteins affect the infected cell by stimulating growth, by causing death, or by inhibiting death so the virus can grow for a longer period of time? Does this vary between variola major and variola minor?
- Do any of the viral proteins provide new potential targets for antiviral drugs that can block virus replication without harming host cells? These targets may suggest new types of drugs that can be developed to treat other infections.

Finally, judging from what is known about other poxviruses, modulation of host immune responses is highly likely to contribute to the virulence of the virus. Infection of immune system cells could make it possible to assess direct effects on such cells, and incubation of human immune system cells with proteins secreted by infected cells could allow identification of potentially unique interactions between viral proteins and mediators of the antiviral immune response. These interactions could be used to identify important and potentially unique aspects of the human response to virus infections.

## VIRUS-HOST INTERACTIONS

Replication of variola virus in different types of cell cultures could provide valuable information on how this virus distinctly infects and affects human cells. It could not, however, provide information on how the virus spreads through the host or how it counteracts the host immune response.

Cultures that involve a number of cells organized into tissues and organs can currently be studied in bioreactors, SCID-hu mice, and raft cultures. These systems could allow investigators to answer some of the following questions:

## UNDERSTANDING OF THE BIOLOGY OF VARIOLA VIRUS

- How does the virus spread from one cell to another in infected human tissue, such as the lung, lymph nodes, and skin? Is this different for variola major and variola minor?
- Does the infection of one cell induce damage or dysfunction in nearby cells, particularly cells of the immune system, without infecting them? What are the viral products and human cell targets for such effects? How does this virus cause such severe damage to human tissues, including inducing encephalitis?

Some questions regarding how the virus spreads and causes immune suppression can be answered only by examining the results of infection in an intact host. Since human infection is not possible, answers to these questions would require developing new animal models (e.g., nonhuman primates, transgenic mice, SCID mice reconstituted with the relevant human cells; see also Chapter 8). With such model systems, the following questions could be addressed:

- How and why does the virus spread so efficiently in human organs?
- How does the virus damage host tissues and cells to cause severe disease? Is this the direct result of virus replication in spleen, lymphoid, and bone marrow cells; virus production of mediators that damage even uninfected human cells; or induction of a harmful antiviral immune response?
- What kinds of effective interventions (antiviral drugs, antibodies, immune modulators) can be developed to treat smallpox or smallpox-like diseases?
- How effective are new types of vaccines?

# 11

# Research on the Expressed Protein Products of Variola

One emerging field in molecular virology is the identification and expression of viral proteins that are not required for the synthesis of new virions, but allow a virus to inhibit or mediate elements of the host immune system [45–49]. Some of these mediatory proteins are very host-specific, while others are not. In most cases studied to date, the viral proteins target unique regulatory or effector components of the immune system. These host immune elements range from the cytokine network, to signal transduction pathways, to complement cascade, to cytotoxic lymphocyte killing mechanisms, to the innate apoptosis response to infections [5, 46, 50]. Of all the mammalian viruses, poxviruses have evolved to encode a larger number of these viral anti-immune molecules than any other virus group [51]. And because variola virus is the only highly pathogenic orthopoxvirus to have evolved in humans alone, its own unique array of anti-immune proteins is believed to be adapted to molecules of the human immune system. Accordingly, there are compelling reasons to predict that expressed variola proteins of this class will exhibit mediatory activities specifically against human immune pathways, only some of which are understood or possibly even as yet discovered.

Viral proteins are generally multifunctional. They form networks—complexes with other proteins, viral and cellular. The functions of these proteins are frequently determined by post-translational modifications (e.g., phosphorylation, nucleotidylation, poly(ADP-ribosyl)ation). A single viral protein expressed in transfected cells may have totally different functions than if expressed in productively infected cells. For example, the localization of herpes simplex virus ICP22 by itself is different from that of the same protein in infected cells. Also, the unphosphorylated protein binds a different set of proteins than the processed (phosphorylated) protein. Live variola virus would be required to verify the function of viral proteins coded by the variola genome.

Sequence information suggests that five kinds of variola proteins could be expressed for research purposes:

• Secreted proteins that function as paracrine ligand mimics, or affect humoral systems such as the cytokine network or the complement cascade.
• Cell surface proteins that mimic cellular receptors or regulate immune recognition molecules, such as MHC-I or CD4.
• Intracellular proteins that regulate cellular signal transduction pathways, such as apoptosis.
• Virion component proteins that can alter immunogenic aspects of the virus particles.
• Proteins that can control or favor the ability of a virus to grow in selected tissues.

Some aspects of variola protein synthesis could be accomplished using only cloned genes, while others would require expression by the live virus. The following sections address first, the kinds of strategies that could be used for synthesis of variola virus proteins, and second, the potential usage of these expressed proteins for the study of human immunology and for the development of novel drugs to treat human immune-based diseases.

## SYNTHESIS OF VARIOLA PROTEINS

All poxviruses have evolved to replicate in the cytoplasm of infected cells and utilize genetic regulatory sequence elements that are virus-specific [52]. Poxvirus messenger RNAs are not spliced, but may contain sequences that preclude efficient expression in heterologous vector systems. In other words, the success of authentic expression of any poxvirus protein in the absence of live virus cannot always be ensured. Some variola proteins can readily be produced in standard expression systems (e.g., bacterial, yeast, baculovirus), but others may be refractory to such expression. In general, there are three major strategies for expressing poxvirus proteins, which differ in their requirements for availability of live variola virus:

• **Expression of single cloned genes.** This strategy utilizes standard expression vectors and requires only cloned variola DNA fragments well characterized in terms of sequence variation. This strategy works only for some poxvirus genes, and does not allow for virus-specific modification events such as post-translational processes under virus control. The strategy also does not facilitate identification of activities that rely on interactions between more than one viral protein or complexes between distinct viral proteins.

- **Co-expression of multiple proteins.** Generally, this strategy requires composite expression vectors or the creation of chimeric viruses that contain larger variola DNA fragments encoding for multiple genes. Given the uniqueness of poxvirus gene regulation, this latter approach would most easily be accomplished with recombinant viruses derived from other poxviruses, such as vaccinia. However, the uncertainty concerning variola genes that determine pathogenesis would mandate strict regulatory restrictions on such recombinant viruses, and it is likely that they would require the same containment and restrictions as live variola virus itself. Moreover, the authenticity of such proteins in comparison with live variola virus would need to be demonstrated.
- **Full genomic expression.** Expression of the full spectrum of variola proteins, which includes all the events of synthesis, post-translational modification, and assembly into potentially active complexes and requires infection of cultured cells with live variola virus. This strategy would probably be the only way to reconstitute variola virus particles for authentic protein functional and structural studies aimed at the analysis of host cell receptors used by the virus or dissemination of the virus through the body.

## POTENTIAL UTILITY OF VARIOLA PROTEINS

The two most important potential uses for variola proteins are as research tools to investigate the human immune system and as a source of new drugs to treat human diseases caused by aberrant immune functions.

First, variola proteins are novel and unique probes of the human immune system. At present, it is estimated that between 10 and 50 percent of the genomic coding capacity of poxviruses is devoted to the expression of proteins that interact with host defense molecules. Many proteins of this class have already been discovered and partly characterized for other poxviruses, with host targets extending across a broad range of immune cell functions. These targets include cytokines (e.g., viral inhibitors of interferon, tumor necrosis factor, interleukin-1); growth factors (e.g., viral mimics of epidermal growth factor, vascular endothelial growth factor); complement (e.g., viral analogs of C4B-binding proteins); apoptosis (e.g., viral inhibitors of the caspase cascade); and various immune cell functions (e.g., viral inhibitors of antigen presentation, macrophage activation or cytotoxic lymphocyte killing mechanisms) [53].

This is an area of active research on many poxvirus systems, and one can only speculate as to how many such anti-immune proteins are expressed by variola virus. As noted earlier, given the long history of variola as an exclusively human-adapted virus, it can be predicted that a substantial number of these viral proteins are targeted to inhibit human immune molecules, some of which undoubtedly remain to be identified. Thus, the expressed variola proteins collectively represent an untapped resource of experimental probes with which it may be possible to identify and characterize new and potentially still-unknown human immune system components.

Second, purified variola proteins might be used as potential drugs to treat human diseases. A number of poxvirus proteins that function to inhibit immune pathways in the context of viral infection also inhibit the same immune molecules when purified and tested in the absence of virus. The discovery and analysis of the biological properties of poxvirus-encoded serpins have yielded a wealth of knowledge about how viruses can modulate inflammation [54]. For example, a secreted serine proteinase inhibitor from a rabbit-specific poxvirus and a similar but different orthopoxvirus homologue of the rabbit-specific poxvirus inhibit human proteinases in vitro [55, 56]. Rabbit poxvirus proteins can prevent inflammatory cell-dependent atherosclerosis in an animal model of vascular restenosis [57]. Similarly, a variety of viral apoptosis, or programmed cell death, inhibitors, such as crmA of cowpox, offer novel avenues for approaching the therapy of diseases associated with excessive cell death [58]. A homologue gene of serp2 found in the rabbit-specific myoxoma poxvirus inhibits some of the molecules involved in controlling apoptosis, but cannot substitute for crmA [59]. Such examples suggest that some viral proteins may be uniquely specific in function. Finally, selected viral proteins from variola could perhaps stimulate immune tolerance pathways, which could lead to improved methods for blocking transplant rejection or achieving increased effectiveness of gene therapy vectors [60].

Although the above uses remain hypothetical, the opportunity to investigate such avenues of research in the future will be dependent on the results of the World Health Assembly vote on the future of variola virus.

# PART IV
♦ ♦ ♦ ♦ ♦

# Findings

# 12

## Summary and Conclusions

Smallpox, caused by variola virus, is a devastating disease with high case-fatality and transmission rates. Inoculation with vaccinia virus is highly protective against natural infection with variola virus. Vaccination, together with the restricted host range and vigilant surveillance efforts, enabled a worldwide containment and inoculation program to eliminate smallpox globally more than 20 years ago. The last case of naturally occurring smallpox was in Somalia in 1977. Known tissue collections containing live variola virus material were subsequently consolidated in two international repositories in the United States and Russia.

Scientific research on live variola virus requires maximum containment facilities. As a consequence, little research on variola has been done since eradication. During that same period, scientific knowledge about the molecular pathogenesis of many viral infections has become considerably more sophisticated through studies of the immunology, virology, molecular genetics, structural biology, and molecular pharmacology of infection. While such investigations enable effective diagnosis, treatment, or prevention of many other viral infections, increased knowledge of variola infection has been limited largely to the cloning and complete sequencing of two strains of variola major from the Asian subcontinent, partial sequencing of one strain of variola major, and one strain of variola minor from Latin America. In addition, a few genes of other strains have been sequenced.

Since the eradication of smallpox, virologists have come to realize that disease-causing viruses are efficient pathogens because of a broad spectrum of mechanisms that can defeat or alter innate defenses or immune system responses. The technologies that have been developed to investigate these phenomena have advanced dramatically in the past 20 years and will almost certainly become even more powerful in the future. As a consequence of these capabilities, novel approaches to biomedical research have emerged. Techniques have been developed to render viruses safer to use in laboratory studies and to provide new animal models with which such studies can be performed. Because variola virus is the only uniquely human orthopoxvirus, it offers the potential for understanding aspects of human biology that may have considerable biomedical significance. Thus variola virus, once considered an agent of human pestilence, may in the future be viewed as a potential source of knowledge and of reagents to support advances in cell biology and immunology. In particular, research using variola virus could assist in understanding the inflammatory response, which is a key process of cell-mediated defense.

In preparation for international deliberations concerning whether all variola virus stocks, stored clinical materials containing variola virus, and live variola virus genome DNA held in the international repositories are to be destroyed, this committee was asked to assess future scientific needs for live variola virus. **The committee was not asked to make a recommendation about destruction or retention of variola virus stocks, and such a determination involves information beyond the purview of the committee.**

## THE BROADER CONTEXT

In carrying out its charge, the committee recognized that the knowledge likely to be obtained from future research using live variola virus must be assessed within a broader context that has changed dramatically since the eradication of smallpox. This broader context encompasses three major global conditions.

First, since the cessation of vaccination programs following the successful eradication of smallpox, the entire global population has become more susceptible to the disease than ever before. Widespread inoculation during the eradication program produced a high level of immunity within the general population that protected those exposed to the virus. A smallpox outbreak occurring today in a highly mobile and susceptible population, in contrast, might spread widely before being recognized and before effective countermeasures could be put in place. If large enough, an outbreak could quickly overwhelm medical response capabilities.

Second, the significant number of individuals in many parts of the world who are immunocompromised as a result of HIV infection, an organ transplant, or chemotherapy limits the potential widespread use of the current smallpox vaccine because it is made from live vaccinia virus. Smallpox vaccination with the vaccinia vaccine, the workhorse of the eradication program, was terminated primarily because of eradication, but also because of concern about rare but serious medical complications that occurred among children with highly compromised cellular immune systems or severe dermatitis. Such problems could be expected to be more prevalent in populations with substantial proportions of immunocompromised individuals.

Third, variola virus is increasingly considered a serious threat as a biological weapon. There is currently concern that the development, production, and stockpiling of weapons based on viruses, bacteria, and fungi have continued. Testimony before a committee of the U.S. Congress, for example, alleged that scientists in the former Soviet Union continued to experiment with these materials on a large scale despite such experiments being outlawed by the Biological Weapons Convention in 1972. Although known stocks of variola virus have been consolidated in two repositories, human tissue and clinical laboratory materials infected with variola virus were widespread before eradication. The high human-to-human transmission rates of smallpox, its devastating medical consequences, and the difficulty of mounting countermeasures all contribute to the attractiveness of variola virus as a terrorist weapon. The probability that variola could reemerge as a threat because of unregistered growth of clandestine virus is an as yet unquantifiable parameter in estimation of the scientific utility of retaining variola virus. Live variola virus would be required for full development of antiviral therapeutics needed to deal with such a threat.

## SCIENTIFIC NEEDS FOR LIVE VARIOLA VIRUS

The committee's charge was restricted to assessment of scientific needs for live variola virus. It did not include consideration of risks that may be associated with retention of the existing stocks, and no attempt was made to determine whether the scientific needs identified by the committee outweigh these risks. Furthermore, the committee did not address the likelihood that the funds and other resources needed to pursue this research, including facilities with suitable biological containment provisions, would be available. It must also be recognized that predicting the future is impossible, and while the committee has done its best to provide an assessment of future scientific needs for live variola virus, the unfolding of actual needs and opportunities is likely to depend on the emergence of unforeseeable technical developments, experimental tools, and model systems. For these reasons, the committee expresses its findings and conclusions below in conditional form: If particular knowledge or capability were to be pursued, would the associated research require live variola virus?

The committee identified six potential areas of research that could require the use of variola virus, and then evaluated for each area whether live virus would be needed for that purpose. Before addressing these six areas, however, the committee notes a need associated with the short-term use of variola virus stocks.

**Genomic sequencing and limited study of variola surface proteins derived from geographically dispersed specimens is an essential foundation for important future work. Such research could be carried out now, and could require a delay in the destruction of known stocks, but would not necessitate their indefinite retention.**

We turn now to the six areas of research examined by the committee with regard to the potential need for live variola virus.

**1. The most compelling reason for long-term retention of live variola virus stocks is their essential role in the identification and development of antiviral agents for use in anticipation of a large outbreak of smallpox. It must be emphasized that if the search for antiviral agents with activity against live variola virus were to be continued, additional public resources would be needed.**

Live variola stocks would have to be maintained if the development of effective antiviral drugs for smallpox therapy and prophylaxis were to be pursued. There is currently no effective antiviral for the treatment or prevention of smallpox. Vaccination, which reduces the severity of the disease if administered within 4 days of exposure, is currently the only recourse for those infected with the disease. Moreover, vaccine supplies have dwindled and may be deteriorating. In addition, as noted earlier, vaccinia vaccine, which is used for smallpox immunization, is a live virus and cannot be used safely with immunocompromised individuals.

Having a number of antiviral agents would provide greater protection against an emergence of drug-resistant variola virus, whether the result of natural evolution or genetic engineering. If new agents were to be developed, cell culture infection assays would be important for demonstrating their activity and effectiveness, and for determining the concentration required to prevent infection or its spread. Some of this testing could be carried out with replication-defective forms of variola virus cultured in cells engineered to complement the defect in the virus. Such replication-defective forms of vaccinia virus have been constructed. Yet other steps in this testing would require the use of live variola virus and recently isolated human cells since measurement of tissue culture activity using other orthopoxviruses or replication-defective forms of variola virus and genetically engineered cell lines could yield misleading results.

Finally, private enterprise has little incentive to undertake the development and testing of agents for smallpox prevention and prophylaxis. Therefore, such studies would be dependent on the availability of public resources.

**2. Adequate stocks of smallpox vaccine would have to be maintained if research were to be conducted on variola virus or if main-**

tenance of a smallpox vaccination program were required. **Live variola virus would be necessary if certain approaches to the development of novel types of smallpox vaccine were to be pursued.**

Vaccinia virus vaccine was effective in eradicating smallpox. As noted earlier, however, current stocks of vaccinia vaccine are limited and may be deteriorating. If it again became necessary to control smallpox with a vaccination program, the current supply would need to be replenished. In addition, if laboratory research using variola virus were to be continued, vaccine would have to be available for laboratory workers, even in the absence of an outbreak.

Retention of live variola virus for vaccine production would not be required if vaccinia vaccine supplies were replenished using established methods of manufacture. Moreover, production of vaccinia vaccines using tissue culture could be pursued without the use of live variola virus. Vaccines derived from tissue culture could be compared with the standard vaccine by evaluation of reactogenicity and immunogenicity (essentially the "take" and immune potency of the vaccine) in human subjects and by laboratory assays. Live variola virus would be required only for testing of novel vaccine development strategies using materials other than live vaccinia virus, such as a DNA vaccine expressing selected variola genes. The above-noted concern about the safety of using vaccinia virus vaccine in populations with high levels of HIV infection or other immunosuppressive conditions is the reason for developing nonstandard vaccines. Since definitive evidence of the protective efficacy of such vaccines could not be obtained in the absence of an outbreak, laboratory testing using live variola virus in as yet undeveloped animal models would be needed for this purpose.

**3. If further development of procedures for the environmental detection of variola virus or for diagnostic purposes were to be pursued, more extensive knowledge of the genome variability, predicted protein sequences, virion surface structure, and functionality of variola virus from widely dispersed geographic sources would be needed.**

Evaluation of the specificity and sensitivity of detection methods for variola virus and other orthopoxviruses would require increased knowledge regarding the DNA sequence not only of variola virus from multiple geographic locations, but also of other orthopoxviruses, especially monkeypox. Development of detection and diagnostic procedures would require field or experimental animal model testing. Such efforts might be carried out using a vaccinia virus with one or more variola virus genes instead of live virus. Although such approaches would be preferable to the use of live virus, current policies prohibit the production and use of recombinant vaccinia virus containing a variola virus gene(s). Moreover, use of recombinants is not likely to fully resolve sensitivity and specificity requirements, because the fidelity of function and level of expression of engineered recombinants may be different from those of variola virus itself. Limited studies with monkeypox virus and the homologous monkeypox protein might be undertaken, however, to confirm the recombinant vaccinia virus data. An adequate database of the abundance and molecular interactions of variola virus surface proteins would enable reasonable comparisons.

Despite residual uncertainty as to whether a surface protein-based detection strategy would work for variola once a sufficient number of variola genomes had been cloned and sequenced and their surface proteins analyzed, the use of live variola virus would not add information worth the risk of exposure to live virus. It may be possible to obtain insight into variations by restriction fragment length polymorphism comparison of variola genes amplified by polymerase chain reaction, but the precise nature of individual gene variation and resultant impact on the protein product(s) requires more detailed sequencing. As noted earlier, sequencing of more variola virus isolates might require a delay in the destruction of known stocks of live virus, but would not necessitate their indefinite retention.

**4. The existence of animal models would greatly assist the development and testing of antiviral agents and vaccines, as well as studies of variola pathogenesis. Such a program could be carried out only with live variola virus.**

The major rationale for testing agents in animal models is to reduce the risk to human subjects and to optimize the design of clinical trials. Given that there is no opportunity to assess the efficacy of agents in infected human subjects short of an outbreak, there would be a serious need for animal model studies if new antiviral agents were to be developed. In the event of an outbreak, moreover, clinical conditions would not lend themselves to rigorous testing of experimental agents. The current absence of suitable animal models for variola virus does not mean that such models could not be developed in the future, given advances in reconstituting certain experimental animals with human genes and cells derived from humans. Virus that had been genetically modified to be defective in its replication could be introduced into animals capable of expressing the needed genes. These and other advances could make testing in animals feasible and safe, and provide protection against a variola virus outbreak.

**5. Live or replication-defective variola virus would be needed if studies of variola pathogenesis were to be undertaken to provide information about the response of the human immune system.**

The specific spatial and temporal patterns of variola virus gene expression must be deciphered in the context of infection at the level of cells, organs, and

# SUMMARY AND CONCLUSIONS

animal models. Studies of these phenomena could provide information on how the virus manipulates the human immune response in order to spread, on the mechanisms of cell death, and on numerous other aspects of variola infection.

**6. Variola virus proteins have potential as reagents in studies of human immunology. Live variola virus would be needed for this purpose only until sufficient variola isolates had been cloned and sequenced.**

Virus-encoded proteins that function as immunomodulators are particularly abundant in poxviruses, and variola virus is uniquely adapted to the human immune system. Thus, it is possible that variola virus could serve as a resource for the discovery of human-specific reagents, including such diverse examples as cytokine inhibitors, anti-inflammatory proteins, and regulators of apoptosis.

Finally, the future scientific needs for live variola virus must be assessed in light of the knowledge that might be derived from studies of other orthopoxviruses, variola virus DNA clones, orthopoxvirus with one or more variola genes, replication-defective variola virus, live variola virus in tissue culture, and live variola virus in animal models. Table 12-1 summarizes this comparison and provides references to more extensive discussion in earlier chapters.

## OVERALL CONCLUSIONS

The most compelling need for long-term retention of live variola virus is for the development of antiviral agents or novel vaccines to protect against a reemergence of smallpox due to accidental or intentional release of variola virus. In addition, much scientific information, particularly concerning the human immune system, could be learned through experimentation with live variola virus.

Indeed, the weight of scientific opinion suggests that continuing investigation of variola virus could lead to new and important discoveries with real potential for improving human health. At the same time, the committee recognizes that limited research infrastructure and resources constrain the realization of this potential. Fortunately, recombinant DNA technology has progressed such that it is now possible to render variola virus incapable of replicating or causing disease. Such genetically crippled variola virus could be used for some steps in the testing of antiviral agents and for some scientific studies.

The risks of retaining the stocks of live variola virus might well outweigh the benefits. If the stocks were retained, however, they could offer the possibility of scientific advances that could not otherwise be achieved.

TABLE 12-1 Potential Scientific Needs for Poxviruses and Their Components

| Research Area | Other Orthopoxviruses | Variola Virus DNA Clones | Orthopoxvirus with One or More Variola Genes | Replication-Defective Variola Virus | Live Variola Virus in Tissue Culture | Live Variola Virus in Animal Models* |
|---|---|---|---|---|---|---|
| Variability of Variola (Chapters 8, 9) | Useful for comparison | Essential | Helpful | Not required | Essential until overlapping and repetitive clones from many isolates are available | Not required |
| Antivirals (Chapter 6) | Helpful | Helpful | Helpful | Helpful | Essential for development steps | Essential for full verification |
| Tissue Culture Vaccines (Chapter 7) | Essential | No use | Helpful | Possible verification | Not required | Essential for full verification |
| Novel Vaccines (Chapter 7) | Helpful | May be used to develop immunogens | Not applicable | Helpful | Helpful for development | Essential for full verification |
| Environmental Detection (Chapter 8) | Essential for early phases | Essential for assessing variola variability | Helpful for field testing | Partial verification | Helpful but not essential | Helpful but not essential |
| Diagnosis of Infection (Chapter 8) | Helpful for determining specificity | Essential | Essential for in vitro or in vivo testing | Helpful but not essential | Helpful but not essential | Helpful but not essential |
| Virus-Cell Interactions (Chapter 10) | Helpful | Helpful | Helpful | Helpful | Essential for some targets | Helpful but not essential |
| Virus-Host Interactions (Chapter 10) | Helpful | Helpful | Helpful | Helpful | Helpful for some targets | Essential for some targets |

*Currently unavailable.

♦ ♦ ♦ ♦ ♦

# References

1. F. Fenner, D.A. Henderson, I. Arita, J. Jezek, and L.D. Ladnyi. *Smallpox and Its Eradication.* Geneva: World Health Organization, 1988.
2. *Encyclopedia Britannica.* "Smallpox" (CD-ROM). 1998.
3. A. Cann. *Principles of Molecular Virology.* London: Academic Press, 1997.
4. K. Alibek. Testimony before the U.S. Congress, Joint Economic Committee. "Terrorist and Intelligence Operations: Potential Impact on the U.S. Economy." May 20, 1998.
5. H.L. Ploegh. Viral strategies of immune evasion. *Science* 280:248–253, 1998.
6. R.F. Massung, V.N. Loparev, J.C. Knight, A.V. Totmenin, V.E. Chizhikov, J.M. Parsons, et al. Terminal refion sequence variations in variola virus DNA. *Virology* 221(2):291–300, 1996.
7. B. Moss. Poxviridae: The viruses and their replication. In B.N. Fields, D.M. Knipe, and P.M. Howley, eds., *Fields Virology.* 3$^{rd}$ ed., Vol. 2. Philadelphia: Lippincott-Raven, 1996.
8. T.G. Senkevich, E.V. Koonin, J.J. Bugert, G. Darai, and B. Moss. The genome of molluscum contagiosum virus: Analysis and comparison with other poxviruses. *Virology* 233(1):19–421, 1997.
9. E.J.H.J. Wiertz, D. Sotorella, M. Bogyo, J. Yu, W. Mothes, T.R. Jones, et al. Sec61-mediated transfer of a membrane protein from the endoplasmic reticulum to the proteasome for destruction. *Nature* 384(6608):432–438, 1996.
10. *Encyclopedia Britannica.* "Viruses: The Cycle of Infection" (CD-ROM). 1998.
11. F. Fenner and R.M.L. Buller. Mousepox. In N. Nathanson, ed., *Viral Pathogenesis.* Philadelphia: Lippincott Raven, 1997.

12. *Encyclopedia Britannica.* "Jenner, Edward" (CD-ROM). 1998.
13. United Kingdom Ministry of Health. Smallpox 1961–63. In *Reports on Public Health and Medical Subjects*, No. 109. London: Her Majesty's Stationary Office, 1963.
14. T. Mack. Smallpox in Europe. *Journal of Infectious Disease* 125(2):161–169, 1972.
15. D.A. Henderson. *Historical Background.* Paper prepared for the Workshop of the IOM Committee on Assessment of Future Scientific Needs for Live Variola Virus, 20 November 1998, Washington, D.C.
16. WHO (World Health Organization). *Report of the Meeting of the Ad Hoc Committee on Orthopox Virus Infections.* Geneva: World Health Organization, 1994.
17. NIH (National Institutes of Health). "Guidelines for Research Involving Recombinant DNA Molecules" (Online). Available at: http://www.nih.gov/od/orda/apndxg.htm. Accessed 15 December 1998.
18. G. Holzer and F.G. Falkner. Construction of a vaccinia virus deficient in the essential DNA repair enzyme uracil DNA glycosylase by a complementing cell line. *Journal of Virology* 71(7):4997–5002, 1997.
19. WHO (World Health Organization). "World Health Assembly Closes in Geneva" (press release). 27 May 1996. Available at: http://www.who.int/inf-pr-1996/wha96-11.html. Accessed October 23, 1998
20. WHO (World Health Organization). Destruction of the smallpox virus. *Weekly Epidemiological Report* (serial online) 74(4):27–28, 29 January 1999. Available at: http://www.who.int/wer/pdf/1999/wer7404.pdf. Accessed 3 February 1999.
21. U.S. Department of Defense/Department of Health and Human Services Smallpox Research Group. *Smallpox Research Plan, Memorandum of Transmittal to National Security Council (Daniel Ponneman)*, 30 June 1995.
22. J. Neyts and E. De Clercq. Efficacy of (S)-1-(3-hydroxy-2 phosphonylmethoxypropyl)cytosine for the treatment of lethal vaccinia virus infections in severe combined immune deficiency (SCID) mice. *Journal of Medical Virology* 41(3):242–246, 1993.
23. K.P. Meadows, S.K. Tyring, A.T. Pavia, and T.M. Rallis. Resolution of recalcitrant molluscum contagiosum virus lesions in human immunodeficiency virus-infected patients treated with cidofovir. *Archives of Dermatology* 133(8):987–990, 1997.
24. J. W. Huggins. Presentation at the Workshop of the IOM Committee on Assessment of Future Scientific Needs for Live Variola Virus, 20 November 1998, Washington, D.C.
25. P.B. Jahrling. Presentation at the Workshop of the IOM Committee on Assessment of Future Scientific Needs for Live Variola Virus, 20 November 1998, Washington, D.C.

26. J.J. Esposito. Comment at the Workshop of the IOM Committee on Assessment of Future Scientific Needs for Live Variola Virus, 20 November 1998, Washington, D.C.

27. E. De Clercq. Antiviral drug discovery. In G.J. Galasso, R.J. Whitley, and T.C. Merigan, eds., *Antiviral Agents and Human Viral Diseases.* Philadelphia: Lippincott-Raven, 1997.

28. *Physicians' Desk Reference.* 52nd ed. Oradell, N.J.: Medical Economics Co., 1998.

29. B.N. Fields, D.M. Knipe, and P.M. Howley. *Fields Virology.* 3$^{rd}$ ed. Philadelphia: Lippincott-Raven, 1996.

30. M.S. Hirsch, B. Conway, R.T. D'Aquila, V.A. Johnson, F. Brun-Vezinet, B. Clotet, et al. Antiretroviral drug resistance testing in adults with HIV infection: Implications for clinical management. International AIDS Society—USA Panel. *Journal of the American Medical Association* 279(24):1984–1991, 1998.

31. B. Mahy and L.Collier, eds. *Virology. Topley and Wilson's Microbiology and Microbial Infections.* Vol. 1. London: Oxford University Press, 1998.

32. CDC (Centers for Disease Control and Prevention). Vaccinia (smallpox) vaccine recommendations of the Immunization Practices Advisory Committee (ACIP). *Morbidity and Mortality Weekly Report* 40(R14):1–10, 1991.

33. R.R. Redfield, D.C. Wright, W.D. James, T.S. Jones, C. Brown, and D.S. Burke. Disseminated vaccinia in a military recruit with human immunodeficiency virus (HIV) disease. *New England Journal of Medicine* 316(11):673–676, 1987.

34. CDC (Centers for Disease Control and Prevention). Epidemiologic notes and reports: Disseminated vaccinia infection in a college student in Tennessee. *Morbidity and Mortality Weekly Report* 31(50):682–683, 1982.

35. CDC (Centers for Disease Control and Prevention). Notice to readers: smallpox vaccine no longer available for civilians—United States. *Morbidity and Mortality Weekly Report* 32(29):387, 1983.

36. S.N. Shchelkunov, R.F. Massung, and J.J. Esposito. Comparison of the genome DNA sequences of Bangladesh-1975 and India-1967 variola viruses. *Virus Research* 36:107–118, 1995.

37. J.J. Esposito. Presentation at the Workshop of the IOM Committee on Assessment of Future Scientific Needs for Live Variola Virus, 20 November 1998, Washington, D.C.

38. R.F. Massung, J.C. Knight, and J.J. Esposito. Topography of variola smallpox virus inverted terminal repeats. *Virology* 211:350–355, 1995.

39. H. Neubauer, U. Reischl, S. Ropp, J.J. Esposito, H. Wolf, and H. Meyer. Specific detection of monkeypox virus by polymerase chain reaction. *Journal of Virological Methods* 74(2):201–207, 1998.

40. M.S. Ibrahim, J.J. Esposito, P.B. Jahrling, and R.S. Lofts. The potential of 5′ nuclease PCR for detecting a single-base polymorphism in orthopoxvirus. *Molecular Cell Probes* 11(2):143–147, 1997.

41. S.L. Ropp, Q. Jin, J.C. Knight, R.F. Massung, and J.J. Esposito. PCR strategy for identification and differentiation of smallpox and other orthopoxviruses. *Journal of Clinical Microbiology* 33(8):2069–2076, 1995.

42. F. Scheiflinger, F. Dorner, and F.G. Falkner. Construction of chimeric vaccinia viruses by molecular cloning and packaging. *Proceedings of the National Academy of Sciences* 89:9977–9981, 1992.

43. P.C. Turner and R.W. Moyer. The molecular pathogenesis of poxviruses. *Current Topics in Microbiology and Immunology* 163:125–151, 1990.

44. R.M. Buller and G.J. Palumbo. Poxvirus pathogenesis. *Microbiological Review* 55:80–122, 1991.

45. G.J. Kotwal. Microorganisms and their interaction with the immune system. *Journal of Leukocyte Biology* 62(4):415–429, 1997.

46. G. McFadden. DNA viruses that affect cytokine networks. In B.B. Aggarwal and R.K. Puri, eds., *Human Cytokines: Their Role in Disease and Therapy.* Cambridge, Mass.: Blackwell Press, 1995.

47. G. McFadden. *Viroceptors, Virokines and Related Immune Modulators Encoded by DNA Viruses.* Austin, Tex.: R.G. Landes Co., 1995.

48. G.L. Smith, J.A. Symons, A. Khanna, A. Vanderplasschen, and A. Alcami. Vaccinia virus immune evasion. *Immunological Reviews* 159:137–154, 1997.

49. M.K. Spriggs. One step ahead of the game: Viral immunomodulatory molecules. *Annual Review of Immunology* 14:101–131, 1996.

50. R.M. Zinkernagel. Immunology taught by viruses. *Science* 271(5246): 173–178, 1996.

51. M. Barry and G. McFadden. Virokines and viroceptors. In D.G. Remick and J.S. Friedland, eds., *Cytokines in Health and Disease.* New York: Marcel Dekker, 1997.

52. B. Moss. Replication of poxviruses. In B.N. Fields, D.M. Knipe, and P.M. Howley, eds. *Fields Virology,* 3$^{rd}$ ed. Philadelphia: Lippincott-Raven, 1996.

53. A.S. Lalani and G. McFadden. Secreted poxvirus chemokine binding proteins. *Journal of Leukocyte Biology* 62, 1997.

54. P.C. Turner, P.Y. Musy and R.W. Moyer. Poxvirus serpins. In G. McFadden, ed., *Viroceptors, Virokines, and Related Immune Modulators Encoded by DNA Viruses.* Austin, Tex.: R.G. Landes Co., 1995.

55. D.A. Lomas, D.L. Evans, C. Upton, G. McFadden, and R.W. Carrell. Inhibition of plasmin, urokinase, tissue plasminogen activator, and C1S by a myxoma virus serine proteinase inhibitor. *Journal of Biological Chemistry* 268(1):516-521, 1993.

56. P. Nash, A. Lucas, and G. McFadden. SERP-1, a poxvirus-encoded serpin, is expressed as a secreted glycoprotein that inhibits the inflammatory response to myxoma virus infection. In F.C. Church, D.D. Cunningham, D. Ginsburg, M. Hoffman, S.R. Stone, and D.M. Tollefsen, eds., *Chemistry and Biology of Serpins.* New York: Plenum Press, 1997.

57. A. Lucas, Y. Liu, J. Macen, P. Nash, E. Dai, M. Stewart, et al. Virus-encoded serine proteinase inhibitor SERP-1 inhibits atherosclerotic plaque development after balloon angioplasty. *Circulation* 94(11):2890–2900, 1996.

58. G. McFadden and M. Barry. How poxviruses oppose apoptosis. *Virology* 8:429–442, 1998.

59. J.A. Macen, K.B. Takahashi, K.B. Moon, R. Nathaniel, P.C. Turner, and R.W. Moyer. Activation of caspases in pig kidney cells infected with wild-type and CrmA/SPI-2 mutants of cowpox and rabbitpox viruses. *Journal of Virology* 72(5):3524–3533, 1998.

60. G. McFadden, K. Graham, and M. Barry. New strategies of immune modulation by DNA viruses. *Transplantation Proceedings* 28(4):2085–2088, 1996.

# APPENDIX A

## Glossary

**Antibody:** An immunoglobulin molecule that has a specific amino acid sequence such that it interacts only with the antigen that induced its synthesis in lymphoid tissue, or with an antigen closely related to it.

**Antigen:** Any substance that is capable, under appropriate conditions, of inducing the formation of antibodies and of reacting specifically in some detectable manner with the antibodies so induced.

**Apoptosis:** A mechanism by which cells self-destruct when stimulated by the appropriate trigger.

**Atherosclerosis:** A common form of arteriosclerosis in which deposits of yellowish plaque containing cholesterol, lipoid material, and lipophages are formed within the large and medium-sized arteries.

**B cell, B lymphocyte:** Bone marrow derived lymphocyte; originally differentiating in bone marrow, it can mature and multiply in the lymphoid organs when suitably stimulated.

**Base pair:** Polynucleotide pairs with each purine base linked to its complementary pyrimidine base in the opposite DNA chain.

**Binding proteins:** Proteins with a high affinity for binding a drug so that its overall potency is reduced and its effect prolonged as a result of its level being maintained in the blood plasma.

**Chimeric viruses:** Viruses into which genes from a different virus have been introduced.

**Chorioallantoic membrane:** A membrane in birds, adjacent to the egg shell, that surrounds the embryo and contributes to gas exchange.

**CrmA gene:** A cytokine response modifier gene that inhibits the proteolytic activation of interleukin-1 beta, thereby suppressing its response to infection.
**Cytokine:** Any of a class of phytohormones whose principal functions are the induction of cell division and the regulation of differentiation of tissue.
**Cytotoxic:** Pertaining to, resulting from, or having the action of a cytotoxin.
**Cytotoxin:** A toxin or antibody that has a specific toxic action on cells of special organs; cytotoxins are named according to the cells for which they are specific.

**DNA:** Deoxyribonucleic acid, a double-helix polymer encoding genetic information for the transmission of inherited traits; comprises two long, linked chains of monomer nucleotides consisting of a deoxyribose sugar molecule to which is attached a phosphate group and one of four nitrogenous bases—two purines (adenine and guanine) and two pyrimidines (cytosine and thymine).
**DNA amplification primer:** A short stretch of nucleotides that bind, or anneal, to the DNA sequence to be cloned and serve as the starting point for copying in a polymerase chain reaction.
**DNA clone:** A DNA fragment produced by propagating and storing a large number of identical molecules having a selected DNA fragment as their single ancestor.

**Enanthem:** An eruption upon a mucous surface.
**Encephalitis:** Acute disease of the central nervous system seen in persons convalescing from infectious disease, usually one of viral origin.
**Epithelial cell:** Surface layer of cells closely bound to one another to form continuous sheets covering surfaces that may come into contact with foreign substances.
**Exanthema:** A condition frequently seen in children, marked by intermittent fever lasting 3 days, falling by crisis, and followed a few hours later by a rash on the trunk.

**Genetic recombination:** The formation of new combinations of genes as a result of crossing over between homologous chromosomes.
**Genome:** A set of chromosomes containing the heritable genetic material that directs gene development.

**Hemagglutinin:** An antibody that agglutinates erythrocytes.
**Hypotension:** Abnormally low blood pressure.

**IgM antibody:** A large immunoglobulin protein with extremely high molecular weight of 19 S.

**IgG antibody:** A large immunoglobulin protein with a molecular weight of 7 S.
**Immunity, active:** Acquired immunity attributable to the presence of antibody or immune lymphoid cells and phagocytic cells formed in response to antigenic stimulus.
**Immunity, herd:** The resistance of a group to attack by a disease because the existing immunity of a large proportion of the members lessens the likelihood that an affected individual will come into contact with a susceptible individual.
**Immunity, passive:** Acquired immunity produced by the administration of preformed antibody or specifically sensitized lymphoid cells.
**Immunogen:** An antigen that can induce antibody production.
**Immunogenicity:** The potency of an immunogen to produce immunity.
**Immunoglobulin:** A protein found in serum and other body fluids and tissues; it functions as a specific antibody that activates humoral aspects of immunity; five classes, based on different antigenic activity, are IgA, IgD, IgE, IgG, and IgM.
**Interferon:** A soluble, small, cell-specific protein that inhibits virus multiplication.
**Intravascular coagulopathy:** A disorder characterized by excessive blood clotting within blood vessels.

**Leukocyte:** A cellular component of blood that helps defend the body from infection by ingesting foreign materials and providing antibodies.
**Lymphocyte:** A type of leukocyte (white blood cell) that is of fundamental importance in the immune system, making up 20 to 25 percent of the total number of leukocytes.
**Lymphokine:** A soluble protein mediator, released by sensitized lymphocytes on contact with antigens, that plays a role in macrophage activation, lymphocyte transformation, and cell-mediated immunity.
**Lysis:** Destruction of cells by a specific antibody.

**Macrophage:** Large phagocytic cells occurring in the walls of blood vessels; usually immobile, they become mobile when stimulated by inflammation.
**Malpighlian layer:** The layer of epithelial cells in the epidermis next to the grain surface of the derma where protoplasm has not yet changed into horny material.
**MHC molecules:** Major histocompatibility complex molecules that are found on the surface of almost all nucleated somatic cells; they control cellular immune reactions and are largely responsible for the rejection of organ transplants.
**Monocyte:** A mononuclear phagocytic leukocyte.
**Morphogenesis:** The development of the structural features of an organism or part.

**Mucous membrane:** Membrane lining body cavities and canals that lead to the outside; chiefly the respiratory, digestive, and urogenital tracts.

**Necrosis:** Death of tissue, usually as individual cells or groups of cells, or in small localized areas.

**Open reading frame:** Two separate additions or deletions of one or two base pairs (reading frame shift) in a DNA sequence such that the second shift restores the reading frame, effectively "skipping" the amino acids coded between the two.

**Papule:** A small, circumscribed, superficial, solid elevation of the skin.
**Paracrine ligand mimics:** Molecules that behave like growth factors or cytokines.
**Pathogen:** Any disease-producing microorganism or material.
**Phagocyte:** Cells that ingest microorganisms or other cells and foreign particles.
**Plasma:** The fluid portion of the blood in which particulate components are suspended.
**Plasmid:** A generic term for all types of intracellular inclusions that can be considered as having genetic functions.
**Polymerase chain reaction:** A technique used to make numerous copies of a specific segment of DNA quickly and accurately; a three-step process carried out in repeated cycles that includes denaturation, or separation, of the two strands of the DNA molecule, each of which is a template on which a new strand is built in the second step, and to which the DNA polymerase adds nucleotides onto the annealed primers in the third step to double the DNA in each cycle.
**Prodrome:** Premonitory symptom.
**Protein:** Any one of a group of complex organic nitrogenous compounds that are the principal constituents of cell protoplasm.
**Pustule:** A visible collection of puss within or beneath the epidermis.

**Raft culture:** Three-dimensional tissue culture, as opposed to a single-layer culture.
**Reactogenicity:** A nonspecific reaction at the site of inoculation, ranging from redness to induration to a lesion or pustule.
**Reading frame:** The set of nucleotide pairs coding for one particular amino acid in the sequence of several thousand nucleotides in a gene; addition or deletion of one or two nucleotide pairs shifts the reading frame from that point to the end of the molecule.
**Reticulum cell hyperplasia:** Overproliferation of stromal cells from certain organs, such as the spleen.

**RNA:** Ribonucleic acid, a complex compound of high molecular weight that functions in cellular protein synthesis and replaces DNA (deoxyribonucleic acid) as a carrier of genetic codes in some viruses.

**Serine proteinase inhibitor:** Protein that blocks the action of host proteases that regulate immunity or inflammation.
**Seroconversion:** Development of antibodies in response to inoculation with a vaccine.
**Serpins:** Serine (crystalline amino acid) protease inhibitor.
**Signal transduction:** Transmission of a signal from one cell to another.
**Subunit protein vaccines:** Vaccines incorporating relevant proteins from a virus instead of the entire virus genome.
**SCID mouse:** Severe combined imunodeficiency mouse, a mouse with a genetic inability to create diversity in its lymphocytes (no functional recombinase gene), so that it lacks an effective immune response; reconstitution with human cells (SCID-hu) can enable the mice to be used to study human diseases.

**T cell, T lymphocyte:** Thymus-derived lymphocyte, referring to lymphatic cell dependency on the maturation process that occurs in the thymus.
**Thymic dysplasia:** Any of a group of hereditary disorders characterized by faulty development of the thymus, which may be associated with normal serum immunoglobulin levels and impaired cell-mediated immunity (Nezelof's syndrome), agammaglobulinemia and impairment of both cell-mediated and humoral immunity, or variable deficiencies of immunoglobulins.
**Titer:** The quantity of a substance required to produce a reaction with a given volume of another substance.
**TNF:** Tumor necrosis factor, a protein produced by macrophages when they encounter the poisonous substance in bacteria known as endotoxin.
**Transgenic:** The property of having genes from other species inserted into the genome.
**Tropism:** The orientation of an organism to an external stimulus.

**Umbilication:** A central, navel-like depression.

**Vascular restenosis:** Narrowing of blood vessels.
**Vesicle:** A small bladder or sack containing liquid; a small blister with circumscribed elevation of the epidermis containing a serous liquid.
**Virion:** The complete viral particle, found extracellularly and capable of surviving in crystalline form and infecting a living cell.
**Viremia:** The presence of viruses in the blood, usually characterized by malaise, fever, and aching of the back and extremities.

# APPENDIX B

♦ ♦ ♦ ♦ ♦

# Acronyms

**BSL-4:** Biological Safety Level 4
**CDC:** Centers for Disease Control and Prevention, Atlanta, Ga.
**CMV:** Cytomegalovirus
**COI:** World Health Organization Committee on Orthopox Infections
**DHHS:** U.S. Department of Health and Human Services
**DOD:** U.S. Department of Defense
**DOE:** U.S. Department of Energy
**EEV:** Extracellular Enveloped Virus
**FDA:** U.S. Federal Drug Administration
**HA:** Hemagglutinin antigen
**HEPA (filters):** High-efficiency particulate air (filters)
**HI:** Hemagglutinin-inhibiting
**HIV:** Human immunodeficiency virus.
**HPMPA:** ((S)-9-(3-hydroxy-2-phosphonylmethoxypropyl)adenine)
**IMV:** Intracellular Mature Virus
**IND:** Investigational new drug
**JCG:** Joint coordinating group
**NIH:** National Institutes of Health
**NYCBH:** New York City Board of Health
**PCR:** Polymerase chain reaction.
**PMEA:** Adefovir, 9-[2-(phosphonomethoxy)ethyl]adenine)
**RLFP:** Restriction fragment length
**UDG:** Uracil DNA glycosylase
**USAMRIID:** U.S. Army Medical Research Institute of Infectious Diseases, Fort Detrick., Md.

**VECTOR:** State Center of Virology and Biotechnology, Koltsovo, Russia
**VIG:** Vaccinia Immune globulin
**WHA:** World Health Assembly
**WHO:** World Health Organization

# APPENDIX C

# Committee and Staff Biographies

**CHARLES C. J. CARPENTER,** M.D. (*Chair*), is Professor of Medicine at Brown University and Director of the Brown University International Health Institute. He is a member of the Institute of Medicine and has held offices in several national professional organizations. He chairs the National Institutes of Health Office of AIDS Research Advisory Committee and the Data Safety Monitoring Board for Clinical Trials of the National Institute of Allergy and Infectious Diseases (NIAID), was a member of the IOM panel on Priorities in Vaccine Development, and has served on numerous scientific advisory committees and panels. He is Program Director of the Centers for Disease Control and Prevention-supported HERS study on the Natural History of HIV Infection in North American Women, Director of the Lifespan/Tufts/Brown Center for AIDS Research, and Chair of the U.S. Delegation of the U.S.-Japan Cooperative Medical Sciences Program, and has served as Chair of the American Board of Internal Medicine and as President of the Association of American Physicians. Dr. Carpenter has received several awards for outstanding contributions to medicine. His M.D. is from the Johns Hopkins University School of Medicine.

**ANN M. ARVIN,** M.D., is Professor of Pediatrics and Microbiology/Immunology at Stanford University School of Medicine. She is a member of the executive committees of the Collaborative Antiviral Study Group of the National Institute of Allergy and Infectious Diseases and of the Varicella-Zoster Virus Research Foundation, and is on numerous editorial and advisory boards; she recently served on the Vaccines and Related Biological Products Advisory Committee, U.S. Food and Drug Administration. Selected recent research publications address the functions of varicella-zoster viral proteins in T cell and skin tropism, immune recognition of structural/regulatory proteins of varicella-zoster virus, early reconstitution of immunity and decreased severity of herpes zoster in bone marrow transplant recipients given inactivated varicella vaccine, and the persistence of humoral and cellular immunity in children and adults immunized with live attenuated varicella vaccine. Dr. Arvin's M.D. is from the University of Pennsylvania.

**R. PALMER BEASLEY,** M.D., is Dean of the University of Texas-Houston Health Science Center School of Public Health and Professor of Epidemiology. He is the recipient of the 1985 King Faisal International Prize in Medicine and the 1987 Charles F. Mott General Motors International Prize for Research on Cancer. Among Dr. Beasley's research accomplishments are studies leading to the understanding of the routes, mechanisms, and timing of the transmission of Hepatitis B Virus (HBV). He helped develop the World Health Organization policy guidelines on HBV immunization and the global HBV control program, and is currently a WHO consultant on HIV and HBV. Dr. Beasley's M.D. is from Harvard University.

**KENNETH I. BERNS,** M.D., Ph.D., is Interim Vice-President for Health Affairs and Dean of the College of Medicine at the University of Florida. He has served as a member of the Composite Committee of the United States Medical Licensing Examination, Chairman of the Association of American Medical Colleges, President of the Association of Medical School Microbiology and Immunology Chairs, President of the American Society for Virology, President of the American Society for Microbiology and Vice-President of the International Union of Microbiological Societies. He is a member of the National Academy of Sciences and the Institute of Medicine. Dr. Berns' research examines the molecular basis of replication of the human parvovirus, adeno-associated virus, and the ability of an adeno-associated virus to establish latent infections and be reactivated. His work has helped provide the basis for use of this virus as a vector for gene therapy. Dr. Berns' M.D. and his Ph.D. in Biochemistry are from The Johns Hopkins University.

**RAPHAEL DOLIN,** M.D., is Dean of the Office for Clinical Programs at Harvard Medical School. He is a past member of the Board of Scientific Counselors of NIAID, the Anti-Infective Drugs Advisory Committee of the U.S. Food and Drug Administration, and the Sub-Specialty Board in Infectious Diseases of the American Board of Internal Medicine. He is past Chair of the Executive Committee of the NIAID AIDS Vaccine Evaluation Group and is currently a member of the NIAID AIDS Research Advisory Committee and the National Institutes of Health AIDS Vaccine Research Committee. His research interests include laboratory and clinical investigation of viral pathogenesis, antiviral chemotherapy, and viral vaccines. Recent publications address analysis of intercurrent HIV-1 infections in phase I and II trials of candidate AIDS vaccines, HIV-1 immunity induced by canarypox, and meta-analysis of five randomized controlled trials comparing continuation of zidovudine vs. switching to didanosine in HIV-infected individuals. Dr. Dolin's M.D. is from Harvard Medical School.

**MYRON E. ESSEX,** D.V.M., Ph.D., is Chair of the Harvard AIDS Institute, Professor of Health Sciences, and Chair of the Department of Immunology and Infectious Diseases at Harvard School of Public Health. He is a member of the Institute of Medicine, and has received numerous awards. He is President of the International Association for Research on Leukemia and Related Diseases, Vice President for Scientific Affairs of the International Retrovirology Association, and member of several scientific advisory boards. Recent publications from his laboratory present evidence that HIV-2 can provide partial protection against subsequent infections of HIV-1 and evidence that African subtypes of HIV-1 have evolved for more efficient heterosexual transmission. Dr. Essex's Ph.D. in Microbiology is from the University of California at Davis.

**DIANE E. GRIFFIN,** M.D., Ph.D., is Professor and Chair of Molecular Microbiology and Immunology at The Johns Hopkins University School of Public Health. She is editor of the *Journal of Virology*, has served on numerous editorial and advisory boards, and is recipient of the Javits Neuroscience Investigator Award. She has participated as a member of the Council of the American Association for the Advancement of Science, the American Society for Virology, and the National Multiple Sclerosis Society, and as Chair of the Microbiology and Infectious Diseases Research Advisory Committee, NIAID. Recent research includes work on measles virus virulence and immune suppression, cytokines in the brain during viral infection, the effect of amino acid changes on alphavirus neurovirulence, and the promotion of functional recovery of alphavirus-infected neurons through preimmunization with nonstructural proteins. Dr. Griffin's M.D. and her Ph.D. in Immunology are from Stanford University.

**ASHLEY T. HAASE,** M.D., is Professor and Head of the Department of Microbiology at the University of Minnesota Medical School. He has been Chairman of the U.S.-Japan AIDS Panel, the AIDS Research Advisory Committee of NIAID, and the Etiology and Pathogenesis Review Panel of the Advisory Panel to the Office of AIDS Research at the National Institutes of Health. He was a Javits MERIT Neuroscience Investigator Awardee (1988–1995) and a NIAID MERIT awardee (1989–1999). Recent publications have addressed genetic evaluation of suspected transient HIV-1 infection of infants, integration of visna virus DNA as a step for productive infection, kinetics of response in lymphoid tissues to antiretroviral therapy of HIV-1 infection, quantitative image analysis of HIV-1 infection, and RNA splice site utilization by simian immunodeficiency viruses derived from Sooty mangabey monkeys. Dr. Haase's M.D. is from the Columbia College of Physicians and Surgeons in New York.

**MARTIN S. HIRSCH,** M.D., is Professor of Medicine at Harvard Medical School, Professor of Immunology and Infectious Diseases at Harvard School of Public Health, and Director of AIDS Clinical Research at Massachusetts General Hospital. He is a member of the Governing Council of the International AIDS Society and has served on numerous editorial and advisory boards. His research interests include the pathogenesis and therapy of human infections with HIV and herpes group viruses. Dr. Hirsch pioneered the use of combination therapy strategies for HIV infection in vitro and in vivo. He is also studying interactions between HIV and CMV, both in vitro and in vivo, and has demonstrated bidirectional potentiation by these viruses. Recent publications address strategies for effective combination antiretroviral therapy for HIV-1 infection in the laboratory and the clinic. Dr. Hirsch's M.D. is from The Johns Hopkins University Medical School.

**ELLIOTT D. KIEFF,** M.D., Ph.D., is Professor of Microbiology and Molecular Genetics and Medicine, Chair of the Virology Program, and Co-Director of Channing Laboratory at Harvard University, and Director of Infectious Disease, Department of Medicine, Brigham and Women's Hospital. He is a member of the National Academy of Sciences and has received many awards, including the outstanding investigator award of the National Cancer Institute. He has served on numerous editorial boards and advisory panels. Recent publications address the molecular pathogenesis of virus-induced malignancies in HIV infection/AIDS, modulation of apoptosis by herpesviruses, and the genetic analysis of Epstein-Barr virus in human lymphocytes. Dr. Kieff's M.D. is from The Johns Hopkins University, and his Ph.D. in Microbiology is from the University of Chicago.

**PETER S. KIM,** Ph.D., is Professor of Biology at Massachusetts Institute of Technology, Member of the Whitehead Institute for Biomedical Research, and Investigator at the Howard Hughes Medical Institute. He is a member of the National Academy of Sciences, a fellow of the American Academy of Microbiology, and a member of the AIDS Vaccine Research Committee of the National Institutes of Health. He has served on numerous editorial and advisory boards and is the recipient of several awards for his scientific work, including the Ho-Am Prize in Basic Science, the DuPont Merck Young Investigator Award of the Protein Society, the Eli Lilly Award in Biological Chemistry of the American Chemical Society, and the National Academy of Sciences Award in Molecular Biology. Selected recent research addresses HIV entry and its inhibition, X-ray crystal structures of the gp41 cores from the HIV and SIV envelope glycoproteins, and the spring-loaded conformational change for influenza hemagglutinin. Dr. Kim's Ph.D. in Biochemistry is from Stanford University.

**BERNARD LO,** M.D., is Professor of Medicine and Director of the Program in Medical Ethics at the University of California, San Francisco. He directs the national coordinating office for the Initiative To Strengthen the Patient-Provider Relationship in a Changing Health Care Environment, which is funded by the Robert Wood Johnson Foundation. He also chairs the End of Life Committee convened by the American College of Physicians, which will develop recommendations for clinical care near the end of life. Dr. Lo is a member of the National Bioethics Advisory Commission and of the Data Safety Monitoring Board for the AIDS Clinical Trials Group at NIAID. His research interests include decisions about life-sustaining interventions, decision making for incompetent patients, physician-assisted suicide, ethical issues regarding HIV infection, and the doctor-patient relationship in managed care. Dr. Lo's M.D. is from Stanford University.

**D. GRANT McFADDEN,** Ph.D., is Professor of Microbiology and Immunology at the University of Western Ontario and Director of Viral Immunology and Pathogenesis Laboratories at the Robarts Research Institute. He has chaired several panels and site reviews for the National Cancer Institute of Canada and is a member of the Poxvirus Subcommittee of the International Committee on the Taxonomy of Viruses. Recent publications address viruses and oxidative stress; inhibitory specificity of the anti-inflammatory myxoma virus serpin, Serp-1; rabbit, hare, squirrel, and swine poxviruses; and viruses and the immune system, Lessons from HIV. He is cofounder of VIRON Therapeutics, a member of the scientific advisory board of VIRON, and a consultant to Gene Chem Management. Dr. McFadden's Ph.D. in Biochemistry is from McGill University.

**BERNARD MOSS,** M.D., Ph.D., is Chief of the Laboratory of Viral Diseases at NIAID and is a member of the poxvirus subgroup of the International Committee on the Taxonomy of Viruses, the National Institutes of Health AIDS Vaccine Selection Committee, and the editorial boards of several scientific journals. He is a member of the National Academy of Sciences and of the American Academy of Microbiology, a Fellow of the American Association for the Advancement of Science, and a past President of the American Society for Virology. Dr. Moss has received numerous awards, including the Dickson Prize for Medical Research and the Taylor International Prize in Medicine. His research focuses on the biology of poxviruses, including virus-host interactions, development of vaccinia virus into an expression vector with application to immune responses to virus infections, live recombinant vaccines, and gene therapy. Dr. Moss's M.D. is from New York University, and his Ph.D. in Biochemistry is from the Massachusetts Institute of Technology.

**RICHARD W. MOYER**, Ph.D., is Professor and Chair, Department of Molecular Genetics and Microbiology, College of Medicine, University of Florida. He serves as Chair of the International Committee for the Taxonomy of Viruses on Poxviruses, as a reviewer for the Department of Defense Poxvirus Branch (AIBS), and as a consultant for the St. Louis University Academic Review Program. He is the recipient of many professional awards and serves on several editorial boards and review panels. Dr. Moyer's research interests include the identification and characterization of genes that contribute to viral (poxvirus) pathogenesis and disease. Recent publications address comparisons among members of the poxvirus T1/35kDa family, nonpermissive infection of insect cells by vaccinia, cytotoxic T lymphocyte assisted suicide, the control of apoptosis by poxviruses, and transient and nonlethal expression of genes invertebrate cells by recombinant entomopoxviruses. Dr. Moyer's Ph.D. in Chemistry is from UCLA.

**HIDDE L. PLOEGH**, Ph.D., is Professor of Immunopathology at Harvard Medical School and Professor of Oncobiochemistry at the Free University of Amsterdam, the Netherlands. He is director of the graduate program in Immunology at Harvard Medical School and is a correspondent of the Royal Dutch Academy of Sciences. He has researched a number of issues of relevance to immunology, in particular MHC-restricted antigen presentation, an area that comprises the interface of immunology and cell biology. Recent publications address stealth strategies used by viruses to escape the host immune system, and more specifically the degradation of Class I MHC molecules catalyzed by human cytomegalovirus gene products. Dr. Ploegh's Ph.D. is from Rijksuniversiteit Leiden, the Netherlands.

**JACK A. SCHMIDT**, M.D., is Senior Director of Immunology and Rheumatology at Merck Research Laboratories. He is Vice-President of the Board of Directors for the Commission on Professionals in Science and Technology, a member of the Minority Affairs Committee of the American Association of Immunologists, and a fellow of the Association for Women in Science. Recent research publications address the structure and function of interleukin-1 beta converting enzyme (ICE), the expression and affinity purification of human inducible nitric-oxide synthase (iNOS), and active-site structure analysis of iNOS with substituted imidazoles. His current research interests include the role of integrins in leukocyte activation and the development of new fluorescence-based technologies with which to measure the subcellular distribution of proteins. Dr. Schmidt's M.D. is from the University of Pennsylvania.

**RICHARD J. WHITLEY, M.D.**, is Vice-Chairman, Department of Pediatrics and Microbiology, and Associate Director for Clinical Studies, Center for AIDS Research, at the University of Alabama at Birmingham. He is past President and current board member of the International Society for Antiviral Research and member of the Council of the International Society for Infectious Diseases. He has edited or co-edited several books, including *Clinical Virology, Antiviral Agents and Viral Diseases of Man*, and *Infections of the Central Nervous System* and has authored or co-authored numerous papers. Recent research addresses issues involving herpes simplex virus, together with application of genetically engineered herpes simplex to treatment of experimental brain tumors; mechanisms, clinical significance, and future implications of viral resistance; and ganciclovir treatment of symptomatic congenital cytomegalovirus infection. Dr. Whitley's M.D. is from The George Washington University School of Medicine.

**FLOSSIE WONG-STAAL**, Ph.D., is Florence Riford Professor of AIDS Research, Departments of Medicine and Biology, University of California at San Diego, and Director, Center for AIDS Research/AIDS Research Institute. She is an honorary member of the American Society of Clinical Investigation and a charter member of the American Society for Virology. She has served on numerous editorial boards and advisory panels. Dr. Wong-Staal's research interests are in the molecular biology of human pathogenic viruses, cancer, and AIDS; mechanisms of gene regulation; novel approaches to gene therapy; and molecular vaccines. Recent publications have addressed advances in gene therapy for HIV and other viral infections, use of ribozymes to inhibit gene expression, and development of HIV vectors for anti-HIV gene therapy. Dr. Wong-Staal's Ph.D. in Molecular Biology is from the University of California at Los Angeles.

## STAFF

**JUDITH R. BALE**, Ph.D., is Director of the Board on Global Health at the Institute of Medicine, which publishes studies that address a range of global issues in biomedical science and science policy. She served for many years with the National Research Council, where she developed and directed international collaborative research projects on specific topics in health and agriculture. She has edited several collections of papers resulting from these programs. She has also directed studies on technology transfer; technological challenges for megacities; population growth and land use change in India, China, and the United States; and international nutrition. Her laboratory research was at the National Institutes of Health and involved enzyme kinetics, structure, and mechanisms. Dr. Bale's Ph.D. in Biochemistry is from the University of Wisconsin, Madison.

**ROB COPPOCK,** Ph.D., is an independent policy consultant and a research associate with the Institute for European, Russian and Eurasian Studies at The George Washington University. He served for many years on the staff of the National Research Council, directed a multiyear international research program on global sustainability, and was Deputy Director of the German-American Academic Council. His current research focuses on global sustainability and climate change. Recent publications address implementation of the Kyoto protocol, comparison of German and American climate change policy, and the use of scenarios in examining regional sustainability. Dr. Coppock's Ph.D. in Economics is from the University of Wuppertal, Germany.